Alcoholism and Problem Drinking

Theories and Treatment

Wes

For Marian

I would like to express my gratitude to John Garcia, Syd Lovibond, Fred Westbrook and Joanna Clarke.

Alcoholism and Problem Drinking

Theories and Treatment

J. Christopher Clarke
with
John B. Saunders

PERGAMON PRESS
SYDNEY • OXFORD • NEW YORK
BEIJING • FRANKFURT • SÃO PAULO • TOKYO • TORONTO

AUSTRALIA	Pergamon Press (Australia) Pty Ltd, 19a Boundary Street, Rushcutters Bay, NSW 2011, Australia
UK	Pergamon Press plc, Headington Hill Hall, Oxford OX3 OBW, England
USA	Pergamon Press, Inc., Maxwell House, Fairview Park, Elmsford, New York 10523, USA
PEOPLE'S REPUBLIC OF CHINA	Pergamon Press, Room 4037, Qianmen Hotel, Beijing, People's Republic of China
FEDERAL REPUBLIC OF GERMANY	Pergamon Press GmbH, Hammerweg 6, D–6242 Kronberg, Federal Republic of Germany
BRAZIL	Pergamon Editora Ltda, Rua Eca de Queiros, 346, CEP 04011, Paraiso, São Paulo, Brazil
JAPAN	Pergamon Press, 8th Floor, Matsuoka Central Building, 1–7–1 Nishishinjuku, Shinjuku-ku, Tokyo 160, Japan
CANADA	Pergamon Press Canada Ltd, Suite 271, 253 College Street, Toronto, Ontario M5T 1R5, Canada

First published 1988

Cover design by Linda Gray

Typeset by Dovatype, Albury, New South Wales
Printed in Singapore by Singapore National Printers Ltd

National Library of Australia
Cataloguing in Publication data:

Clarke, J. Christopher.
Alcoholism and problem drinking.

Bibliography.
Includes index.
ISBN 0 08 034433 X

1. Alcoholism—Treatment. 2. Alcoholics—Rehabilitation. 3. Behavior modification. I. Title.
616.86'106

Contents

On the vexing question of terminology we have abandoned attempts at she/he and he/she combinations and chosen to refer to therapists and patients alike as 'he' and 'him'. We hope that this will not be misconstrued as an endorsement of sexist language. In the choice between 'client' and 'patient' we have decided in favour of the latter, although we acknowledge that the word has unfortunate associations in that it suggests the passive role of a person seeking help. Our belief is that the person seeking assistance should be an active partner in the therapeutic process.

Foreword

> Induction has been practised from morning till night by every human being since the world began. The man who infers that mince pies disagreed with him because he was ill when he ate them, well when he ate them not, most ill when he ate most and least ill when he ate least, has employed, unconsciously but sufficiently, all the tables of *Novum Organum*.
>
> Thomas B. Macaulay, 1860, *Essays*

Macaulay could hardly have picked a better case to reduce Frances Bacon's ostentatious tables of induction to mundane routine. Relating tainted food to gastric upset is even more pedestrian than Macaulay knew, for that logic must have been practised by the lowly gastropod before the lordly *Homo sapiens* appeared on earth. A food-nausea programme was hard-wired in the medulla of the ancient catfish and embedded in the brain stem of the salamander, the first vertebrate to set foot on land. The homologue of this prehistoric piscine system for adjusting the palatability of food commensurate with its effect on the gut can be found in all birds and mammals including, of course, human beings.

In this excellent volume Clarke and Saunders bring together information from different disciplines and a great variety of sources in their analysis of alcoholism. However, nothing captures better the idea they express of the interplay of psychology, medicine and biology than the workings of this system.

The neural logic system works both ways; any flavour followed by gut malaise tastes 'bad' next time it contacts the mouth and any flavour followed by nutritious repletion tastes 'good' when it is encountered again. The mechanism co-evolved in the interplay between herbs and herbivores as the plants instituted chemical defences against foragers and the animals, in turn, developed chemical receptors to circumvent poisons and obtain nutritious fodder. Ultimately, symbiotic relationships may evolve as the plant feeds the animal while the animal assists the plant to pollinate and disperse its seed. For example, such mutual relationships exist between yucca moths and yucca plants and between humans and corn.

Macaulay erred if he implied that rejection of mince pie depends upon a cognitive process in which the subject is aware of his gastric illness, remembers the mince pie and recalls past occasions when the amount of mince pie consumed was correlated with the intensity of gut malaise. In fact, the human subject may fall fast asleep and his illness may come and go before he wakes leaving him without memory of its passing, yet when that subject encounters mince pie again, it will taste 'bad' and he will be at a loss to explain his newly acquired distaste for his favorite dessert. This particular form of 'sleep learning' has been verified experimentally many times over. In the behavioural laboratory after drinking a sweet harmless substance, a rat put under deep anaesthesia and injected with a brief-acting emetic chemical, will reject that sweet fluid when it is offered several days later. In the neurophysiological laboratory the excised oral receptors and buccal ganglia of the garden snail will acquire a food-toxin aversion *en vitro*. The unconscious rat and the neural apparatus of the snail display the same degree of 'intelligence' in solving the flavor-nausea problem as that exhibited by either Frances Bacon or Thomas Macaulay.

The analysis of ingestive habits indicates that the classic CS-UCS formula should be expanded to include this unconscious motivational process as well as a cognitive learning process (for instrumental conditioning simply substitute 'response' for CS and 'reinforcer' for UCS in the following formulation):

CS (cue)–UCS (flavour)——Feedback (gut)

The CS–UCS association is primarily the result of cognitive processing. The subject driven by hunger or thirst is aroused and learns about the contiguencies between distal CS cues and the flavour UCS of food or drink in the mouth. According to Edward C. Tolman, the subject acquires a 'cognitive map' of what leads to good (or bad) flavours in the context of time and space and modifies his motor behaviour accordingly. The same sort of cognitive mapping strategies enable him to seek comfortable shelters and avoid painful insults to skin. Conscious awareness and brief CS–UCS intervals facilitate the acquisitions of effective cognitive maps. But US–FB integration is an entirely different matter; it is a motivational process which adjusts the hedonic value of flavour according to its utility in the internal economy of the gut. It can operate effectively over long US–FB intervals without awareness or memory of any relevant spatiotemporal cognitive map. As Sigmund Freud taught, a half century ago, we are rarely aware of the source of our motives. Thus Macaulay was perhaps more accurate than he knew, when he implied the devaluation of mince pie was 'unconscious'.

The incentive modification system for food evaluations is distinct from, but interconnected with, the instrumental-motor system for obtaining food and protecting the skin from predatory attacks. The two systems display reciprocal inhibition as the animal allocates time and energy to one function or the other. If the animal eats a large meal it usually retreats to a safe place where the instrumental-motor system relaxes, sleep ensues and the incentive-modification of the meal flavour proceeds even as the animal sleeps. However if the meal is followed by stress exciting the motor system gastric stasis ensues and incentive modification is inhibited. Thus failure can occur, but under the natural rhythms of the world in which we evolved the dual systems operate reasonably well.

The authors of this book are aware that the interaction of our herditary nature with the world of high technology is very apt to cause 'illogical' behaviour and that simplistic behaviour modification programmes can backfire in unexpected directions. For example, when warning a laboratory subject that food or drink is poisoned, loud auditory and bright visual alarms are ineffective but a slight taste or a faint odour will work wonders. Shocking the subject to the feet, or to the mouth for that matter, will cause the subject to consume more, not less, of the forbidden substance in the future. Pinching the rat's tail or forcing it to wait for food will cause it to drink copious amounts of nasty fluids that it would reject under ordinary circumstances. The authors know that the quality of warning signals and punishments must fit the nature of the beast as well as the specific behaviour to be eliminated.

Seeking altered states of awareness for pleasure, we utilize refined and concentrated substances manufactured in legal and illicit laboratories, often irreparably damaging internal organs and addicting our brains. Long ago Edward Thorndike explained this self-destructive behaviour, suggesting that substances such as tobacco, alcohol and morphine reward the controlling neurons of our brain while destroying the cells of our entire body. He said that we are not 'completely adapted' to such substances. Clarke and Saunders offer programmes for a more complete adaptation to the spiny thickets of civilisation; programmes founded on our evolutionary history and our inherent biology, and tested by a vast accumulation of experimental data.

John Garcia

CHAPTER 1

Alcohol Problems: An Overview

Excessive alcohol consumption is the second largest preventable cause of death in the Western world (the first being smoking). Prevalence data are difficult to fix precisely and there are differing standards currently in use for establishing the existence of problem drinking. In addition, there is the tendency for people to underestimate their alcohol intake. Allowing for all of these distorting influences, the most reliable figures for Australia, the United States and Canada show that 80 per cent of adults drink alcohol and one in seven of them can be classified as a problem drinker.[1] The adverse consequences of excessive drinking extend into every sphere of life—medical, psychological and social. There are ample statistics which could be quoted at this point, but none more striking than this: at any point in time the number in the problem drinking population receiving clinical assistance, of any kind, is in the vicinity of 10 per cent or lower.[2] The figure might be less alarming if alcohol problems diminished over time, without counselling or therapy. Disorders that do so are said to have a high rate of 'spontaneous remission' (for example, depression). Alcohol problems, however, do not have a high rate of untreated 'cures': the spontaneous remission rate is thought to be below 20 per cent, possibly as low as 5 per cent (depending on the drinker's age, level of dependence, and other factors).[3] Given the personal, social and economic costs of chronic excessive drinking it is astonishing that nine out of ten problem drinkers go untreated. In the light of the following summary statistics on the consequences of excessive drinking, the very low treatment rate could be considered a social catastrophe.

1. Alcoholics have a mortality rate 250 per cent higher than non-drinkers and the life span of the chronic excessive drinker is shortened by up to 12 years.[4]
2. It is well known that in 50 per cent of all motor vehicle acci-

dent fatalities alcohol is a significant factor, but it is not as widely publicised that upwards of 40 per cent of all pedestrians struck by vehicles have a blood alcohol level themselves in excess of the legal limit for driving.[5]

3. Of all those attempting suicide, 65 per cent had been drinking at the time of the attempt.[6] While this does not prove that the alcohol they consumed caused the attempts, there is a well-established link between drinking and depression, and no one knows how much alcohol it takes to shift an attitude of desolation into an attempt at suicide. Whatever the precise nature of the link, it has been shown that half all suicides are committed by alcoholics[7] and the rate of suicide among problem drinkers is 55 times greater than in the general population.[8]

An exhaustive list of the damage and misery associated with the habitual consumption of alcohol would fill volumes: the few statistics just listed are sufficient to make the point. Why do so many of the millions with alcohol problems escape recognition until their drinking has reached dangerous levels, or until catastrophic consequences ensue? What stands in the way of accurate detection and early, successful treatment? Working on the assumption that there are no barriers to detecting alcoholism, therapists and investigators have focussed their attention on the search for remedies. This confidence in the easy identification of problem drinking is now under challenge.

Contributing to this false confidence are several misconceptions and questionable assumptions about the significance of alcoholism to society when compared with the use of 'hard' drugs like heroin, and about the kinds of people who succumb to it. Of these, perhaps the most pervasive in Western societies is the belief that illicit ('hard') drugs pose a greater threat to the individual and to the community than does alcohol. It is held that there are 'good' drugs ('a nice cold beer'; 'a fine vintage wine') and 'bad' drugs (marijuana, heroin, cocaine). Examples of this neat and comforting dichotomy can be found in media treatments of 'the drug menace'. As an example, there is the story in *Time* magazine (July, 1986) on 'Drugs and Death', the centrepiece of which was a graph superimposed on a drawing of a skull. The graph indicated the number of Americans who have died from cocaine use in recent years, the message being that cocaine, which has replaced heroin as the media drug-of-the-month, is responsible for an epidemic of physical and psychological problems occurring now in the United States. The figures actually showed a forecasted rise in cocaine fatalities from 560 in 1985 to 580 in 1986. That same number, 580, is the amount of alcohol-related fatalities that occurred in the US in 1986 by mid-day on January 3, with the count starting at midnight on New Year's Day. Similar enormous disparities are evident in the Australian figures. Using the most recent data, the estimated number of deaths per year is 200 from heroin and between 4000 and 8000 for alcohol.[9] If we take figures for those in trouble with 'hard' drugs and with 'social' drugs, we again see a glaring disparity between the number of 'alcohol problems' and 'drug problems'. In the US the ratio of alcohol abusers to heroin users is estimated to be in the order of 40 to 1. The figure for alcohol abusers is in all probability higher since it is easier to hide alcohol-related deaths.

Tyler's[10] opening remarks in his 1985 book on drug problems express his (and our) astonishment at the evaluation by Western societies of what are and what are not acceptable ways of using chemical substances to alter mood. 'For anyone caught in possession of a joint (of marijuana) or for that matter a wrap of heroin the special, almost exalted place alcohol occupies . . . will be a perpetual irritant. What other drug can floor a full-grown man within half an hour, is as freely available, so freely advertised and dressed up not as a drug—with all the concomitant health implications—but as a happy social lubricant.' The author is not calling for a repetition of that tragicomic period of Prohibition which failed so disastrously in 1920s America. What he is saying, simply, is that to penetrate our personal and social defences, alcohol must be seen for what it is: a drug which can maim and kill.

The underestimation of the number of problem drinkers and the consequences of the overuse of alcohol are not confined to the media. Recently published generalist texts in psychology and psychiatry continue to give a disproportionate amount of space to the illicit drugs when compared with the attention paid to alcoholism (and smoking). In the latest (1984) edition of Rosenhan and Seligman's volume on abnormal psychology, the amount of space devoted to heroin was more than double that given to alcoholism. We do not wish to single out these authors for special criticism: it is precisely because their book is one of the best available that their unbalanced coverage is so particularly distressing. The 1985 edition of Kaplan and Sadock's *Modern Synopsis of Comprehensive Psychiatry* does give more reference to alcoholism, but also devotes additional space to opiate (for example, heroin) dependence.

Directly related to the high miss rates is the long-standing belief in the existence of dramatic and unmistakeable behaviour patterns and personality characteristics in people with serious drinking problems. The clinical and social stereotype of 'the alcoholic' identifies him as a psychologically weak individual who becomes 'addicted' to alcohol because of the escape from the pressures of life which drinking affords. Out-of-control drinking quickly and inevitably eventuates, followed by social and physical disintegration, with the alcoholic finally 'hitting bottom' and drifting into a Skid Row existence. Such people, it is thought, are easy to identify by their derelict status and a life-style which revolves around getting enough liquor to stay drunk for as long as possible.

Skid Row drinkers constitute about 5 per cent of all problem drinkers and yet the belief in the existence of a readily detectable at-risk population of alcoholics persists. Adherence to this belief is a virtual guarantee that the 'ordinary' drinker presenting with an alcohol related problem will receive enough assistance to manage the symptoms of alcohol abuse (work problems, depression, bones broken in falls, and so on) while his problem drinking is ignored. In a study by Blane and his associates[11] on the vigilance for possible alcohol problems in emergency wards, not one patient was questioned or diagnosed outside the area associated with the presenting injury. This despite the fact that signs of alcoholism were either manifestly present or heavy drinking was the direct cause of their emergency. In another American study Blane, Overton and Chafetz found evidence for an expectancy to encounter a collection of (spurious) 'social factors' in their assessments for the presence of alcoholism. Blane[12] and his team examined the large number of missed cases and discovered that clinicians attached little significance to the social-psychological factors influencing the patients' actions. Blane et al. were struck by 'the [clinicians]' tendency to see alcoholism as a disorder that occurs primarily among socially isolated and impoverished chronic inebriates'. Hore[13] also commented on the clinical costs of this blinkered understanding of drinking problems: 'It means that the "end state" of alcoholism becomes the only form recognized'.

Blane[14] found that the cases missed were more likely to show none or few of the characteristics of the 'Skid Row' drinker. The problem of false negatives means that front-line counsellors have to break free of the 'Lost Weekend' image of alcoholism and come to see 'that the alcoholic in the early stages . . . is hidden and in social terms not very different from his non-alcoholic peers'.

Until this is understood alcoholics will continue to be stigmatised as poor prospects for treatment. The unquestioned and widespread pessimism about the treatment of alcoholism makes sense if we implicitly confine the term to those drinkers who are almost by definition 'bad bets'. To see how this self-fulfilling prophesy is maintained, one fact and one misconception can be put together. The great proportion of problem drinkers are not detected until the drinking and attendant difficulties have become severe and therefore obvious. The 'Skid Row' misconception tends to discourage early cases from receiving treatment and 'particularly among [doctors] will create therapeutic pessimism'.[15] This is, of course, to be expected. If the majority of cases encountered in a clinic falling into a particular diagnostic category are, invariably, 'difficut customers' then a vicious cycle is set in motion. Since it mixes a fallacy (Skid Row) with a fact (end-stage drinkers are poor prospects) the effect is especially pernicious. In the 1960s Trice[16] found that '[T]reatment personnel such as nurses, social workers and doctors frequently view the alcoholic as an undesirable patient and are generally reluctant to treat him'. At the start of the 1980s Jacobs[17] found the same negative expectancies and pessimism. 'On the whole, members of the helping professions . . . view the effect of their work with pessimism and frequently admit that they would prefer to work with clients whose prognoses are more favourable. Many look upon their helping role with what can best be described as a sense of resignation.'

The fault lies with the appealingly simple but demonstrably wrong assumptions that 'real' alcoholics come from the population of derelicts, the unemployed or the lowest socio-economic levels, and are untreatable. These assumptions must be rejected, along with the belief that there is one, correct, treatment for all problem drinkers.

Excessive consumption of alcohol is *the* drug problem in our society. At the same time, the overwhelming proportion of those who regularly drink to excess escape the attention of non-specialist clinicians. Those drinkers who are spotted often refuse treatment, especially if it requires them to concede to the label of 'alcoholic'—a label which they are told they must accept. To add to this unhappy state of affairs, the treatments offered are too often administered by sceptical clinicians. The myths and misconceptions which flourish cause and justify their pessimism. This situation is tragic and unnecessary.

CHAPTER 2

The Disease-Abstinence Model: A Critical Analysis

A review of treatment outcomes for problem drinkers covering the last 30 years reveals two distressing collections of findings: of those drinkers who concede the existence of a problem and request help, most do not improve and, of the small percentage who do, more than half return to practices of harmful drinking. While there is no dearth of treatments on offer, what is to be made of their claims of effectiveness is another matter. For the most part, scientific evidence for their value is non-existent, a state of affairs that has not deterred their adherents from giving them dogmatic support.

Of late, treatments for drinking problems have begun to undergo substantial change: new therapies and novel applications of old techniques are being reported in the specialist journals. To date this information remains largely sequestered in technical publications, with the result that practitioners in medicine, psychology and the other helping professions are largely unaware of these changes, or of the underlying theoretical shifts in thinking about alcoholism. The inaccesibility of the material is not the only obstacle to the application of these findings. Even if some way were found to make this information readily available to the practicing clinicians who would benefit from it, it is by no means certain that it would be accepted. The field of alcohol studies and, most especially, the area of treatment, is highly controversial. While some practitioners might wish to leave the arguments to others and devote their energies to clinical practice, such a stance would leave them ignorant of the changing orientation to theory and research data which have supported some and invalidated other 'commonsense' traditional treatments.

Of the many approaches to theory and practice in the field of alcoholism, two contrasting explanations have dominated. They are the medical-disease model and the learning-conditioning model. In terms of overall influence the two are by no means equally balanced. The former is much more widely favoured, but support for the learning-conditioning model is growing. A brief history will help to establish the necessary context for a discussion of an emerging position which differs from both.

Following in the wake of Prohibition and the Temperance Movement, Alcoholics Anonymous, a self-help organisation with a membership of ex-drinkers, was established just prior to the Second World War. At about that time, in 1937, the influential Yale Centre for Alcohol Studies was set up under the leadership of E.M. Jellinek. Professor Jellinek did as much as any person to legitimise the idea of alcoholism as a disease. One of the principal aims of the Alcoholics Anonymous movement, Jellinek and their allies was to promote, as a deliberate tactic, the idea of alcoholism as a medical disorder 'to combat stigma and prejudice and to improve the image of the [problem drinker] among the helping professions. It was also intended to distance the alcoholic from other groups with much more spoiled identities such as drug addicts and the mentally ill'.[1] This separation, a radical step in its time, continues today as the conventional wisdom. Throughout the Western world there are 'drug and alcohol' authorities, commissions, task forces and the like which, in the names given them, make a subtle and questionable distinction that divorces alcohol problems from the 'serious' drug disorders. This is a distinction which flies in the face of well-documented findings on the injury and mortality rates from the excessive use of alcohol versus the much lower rates for all other drugs combined, which include heroin, cocaine, and 'crack' (but exclude cigarettes, the other 'non-drug' drug).

Moral model and medical/disease-abstinence model

Whatever the shortcomings of the medical/disease-abstinence model, it represented an advance over the model based on the stern Christian morality which it supplanted (although not completely). In the moral model the alcoholic is seen as a spiritually weak person who yields to temptation, with no other thought than for his own selfish and sinful gratification.

With the advent of the medical/disease-abstinence model, the alcoholic was accorded the protection of the sick role, which, understandably, the manufacturers of alcoholic drinks endorsed wholeheartedly. As seen through the focus of this model, alcoholism was caused by a physical defect: the problem was within the alcoholic, rather than within the drink. This was all the ammunition the alcoholic drink producers needed to fight the members of the Temperance Movement, who were vociferous in condemning all consumption of alcohol and its ready availability.

The shift to the medical model took place in the early part of the twentieth century when medical science was coming into maturity. It had been discovered that syphilis, once taken as a symptom of a psychological disorder, had an organic basis and responded to physical treatments. This was taken by the medical profession as a model for the explanation of all emotional and behavioural problems. Alcoholics Anonymous (AA) helped to establish this way of thinking about alcoholism in all of the helping professions and by the general public. At the time AA filled a void caused by the neglect of alcohol problems in medicine and psychology. This neglect was due mainly to the failure to detect the better prognosis early-stage drinkers from those drinkers whose long-term intake of alcohol had put them in the poor prognosis category. When no one else cared to extend a hand to people with serious alcohol problems, members of AA gave counsel and support. For alcoholics with nowhere else to turn, their willingness to make middle-of-the-night visits and the unstinting fellowship they gave to 'dry alcoholics' made the difference between recovery and a shattered life or an early death.

The attraction of AA is due in no small part to the directness and simplicity of its philosophy. AA gives two reasons for long-term abusive drinking or alcoholism, (the terms being synonymous in AA): an 'obsession' and an 'allergic' reaction to alcohol. In common parlance the word 'allergy' is taken to mean a painful or irritating reaction to a particular substance, but as used by AA it means an irresistible pull towards alcohol, a craving rather than a rejection. It is an unquestioned belief that the 'allergy' is activated *automatically* and *immediately* drinking begins. Once activated, the drinker is unable, of his own accord, to refrain from further consumption. Drinking will cease only when the alcoholic loses consciousness, runs out of money to purchase more alcohol or is forcibly restrained from further drinking. The 'allergy' is why the person drinks out of control *after the first drink*. The drinking begins again the next day, and continues the following day because the alcoholic is in the grip of an 'obsession of the mind'.

This 'obsession', something akin to a malignant delusion, is a conviction in the drinker that, regardless of his past history, he will be able to keep his intake of alcohol down to safe, reasonable limits.

A concise statement of this core position of AA on the drinker's dilemma, first articulated in 1939 and held as tenaciously today by its members and allies, is the one expressed in its 'Bible', *Alcoholics Anonymous*: 'The idea that somehow, someday he [the drinker] will control and enjoy his liquor is the great obsession of every abnormal drinker. The persistence of this illusion is astonishing. Many pursue it into the gates of insanity or death'. In their comment on this position critics have consistently noted the implications of the AA philosophy: 'The "allergy" conceptualization put forward by AA not only implies that "alcoholism" is a distinct entity which can be described and recognised despite its variation, but also assumes that certain individuals (alcoholics or pre-alcoholics) have a biological predisposition toward alcohol problems'[2] while other drinkers do not. The AA position, as stated in their publication is: 'The action of alcohol on [those with the disease] is a manifestation of [the] allergy ... [T]he phenomenon of craving [for alcohol] is *limited to this class and never occurs*' in other drinkers; 'these alcoholic types can *never safely use alcohol in any form at all*' (emphasis added).[3]

Perhaps the most widely known and accepted statement from AA about excessive drinkers is contained in these well-known words: 'Once an alcoholic, always an alcoholic'. Years of sobriety will not alter that fact. An abstainer is given the status of 'dry alcoholic', but he must acknowledge that he is, and always will be, an alcoholic.

Orthodox clinical views

AA is not formally affiliated with medical associations, or professional groups, but the commonalities between the views of orthodox clinicians and the disease-abstinence model of AA is undeniable. Here are three representative examples of the AA view from widely-published medical practitioners:

> 'He [the problem drinker] must stop drinking ... I have learned that he will not stop until he gets into an Alcoholics Anonymous program that will enable him to get control of his life without [any] alcohol ... There is no other worthwhile

> treatment; alcohol is too powerful. Alcoholics Anonymous is the only program that I know of that helps . . . [it is] probably the best we have available'[4].

The second is from a leader in the psychoanalytic movement which does not subscribe to a disease model of alcoholism, postulating instead a mental rather than a physical disorder underlying drinking problems. Excessive drinking is explained as a symptom of a personality disorder which takes the form of an unconscious conflict between powerful but socially unacceptable psychosexual urges and defences against these impulses:

> 'When the propitious time arrives an explanation must be given to the patient of how alcohol is poisonous to him (in *any* amount) because *he has built up an allergy to it.* It must be stressed that he is different from other persons and for this reason he is unable to tolerate alcohol.
>
> The patient must abandon the prevailing idea, so current amongst alcoholics, that eventually he will get to a point where he can drink like everyone else. He must be assured that one drink is equivalent to 1000 . . . [H]e must make up his mind to forsake drink completely'.[5]

The third is from a popular book written by a Canadian physician entitled *Alcoholism: A Treatable Illness*: 'The first drink [by the alcoholic] triggers a chain reaction which he or she is powerless to control'.[6]

The disease-abstinence model is stated in the same terms by writers of diverse backgrounds, directly or indirectly implicating a psychophysiological derangement within the alcoholic. In contrast, the learning-conditioning model developed in the 1960s denies any relevance to biological causes at any stage in the development of problem drinking. It states that culture, upbringing and conditioning tell us why drinking becomes a problem, and the laws of learning supply the conceptual and technical tools to lower it to moderate levels. There is no logical reason why those who espouse the environmentalist position should pay so little attention to the desirability of abstinence goals in therapy, except perhaps that since the attainment of controlled drinking is possible for some it must be possible for all. A third and more complex model of alcoholism which contains ideas borrowed from both these extremes is now beginning to take shape, but the disease-abstinence model is still by far the stronger of the two.

The disease-abstinence model in the media

' "This one is ready to go home. . ."

"And what will happen?" [Asks the visitor of the attending physician.] "Will he start all over again?"

"Possibly," [answers the doctor.] "They usually do. But that is something beyond our control. Most of them come back again and again . . . There isn't any cure besides just stopping [completely] . . . You and I do not realize it but liquor does not mean to us what it does to them." '

This passage is from Charles Jackson's novel *The Lost Weekend*, published over 50 years ago, which became a best-seller and later a powerful film which carried the disease-abstinence model to the general public. It was so influential that the book's title passed into the lexicon to signify the out-of-control alcohol bender. Commonly-held ideas about alcoholism have remained virtually unchanged since this book and the film came out. They are stated over and over with little variation, as in a feature article that appeared in 1986 in the popular American magazine *Harpers* by a self-described alcoholic: 'The "ism" alcoholism is a disease . . . We drunks are all sailors stumbling and reeling from tavern to tavern . . . We see the drunkard lifting himself from the bottom time and again only to slip back.' It contains the usual appeal for drinkers to make a commitment to AA and total abstinence: 'In AA we dry moist souls.'

The clinicians' disease-abstinence model and popular conceptions of alcoholism have different starting points but both rest on these axioms:

- There are two quite different types of drinkers: alcoholics and all others. ('Liquor doesn't mean to *us* what it does to *them*.')
- The only way to arrest the disease is to stop drinking alcohol for ever. ('There isn't any cure besides just stopping.')
- The disease cannot be cured, only arrested (in the manner of diabetes) by a rigid unwavering sobriety. If a drink is taken, regardless of how small the amount, or how long the dry period has been, the full-blown syndrome and all of the associated disorders will re-emerge. Drinking will inevitably become out of control ('Most of them come back again and again').

A critique of the disease-abstinence model

Defenders of the disease-abstinence position insist that abstinence is the goal towards which all therapies must aim. The 'disease' referred to is used solely to back up the loss-of-control theory. Critics of this model miss the mark when they concentrate their attacks on the failure of researchers to locate the presumed biochemical defect which constitutes the disease.

The absence of evidence for a disease process bringing about problem drinking has not stopped those who hold the model from attacking claims that some problem drinkers, at least, can learn to moderate their drinking through acquiring the skills of stress management and self-control. Old ideas about alcoholism are treated as modern wisdom—a wisdom which appears impervious to contradictory evidence, whatever the source. If evidence is produced to show that some alcoholics can acquire patterns of normal drinking the reply is to claim that all who did so could not have been true alcoholics in the first place.[7] The way out of this circular reasoning is to subject the tenets of the disease-abstinence model to critical scrutiny, in order to discover its strengths and weaknesses. Once this has been done the task will then be to establish the best possible answers to the causes of chronic excessive drinking and the best possible remedies.

Tenet 1: alcoholism is a disease

Detractors scoff at the idea of alcoholism being a disease: 'If alcoholism is a disease, it is the only one that you can purchase at a store.' This criticism both misses the point and makes the very error that it condemns by implying that a disease resides within the body, unaffected by external circumstances. Not even a medical theory fully committed to the biological bases of all psychological disorders would deny that what the patient does can influence the course of the disease he 'has'. Diabetes provides a case in point. It is a disease (of the pancreas) but it can be controlled if the patient behaves responsibly and takes insulin every day: it can be fatal if he eats sweets whenever he feels the urge to do so.

A disease is not an autonomous process that resides within the skin, unaffected by emotions, behaviour or lifestyle. A disease is a convention which has value to the extent it sheds light on the origins of a disorder, its prognosis and its response to treatment.

It is an open question as to whether problem drinkers should be considered diseased, in any meaning of the word. Even if evidence comes to light that excessive drinking is a disease—and none has yet—that would not rule out environmentally-based interventions, nor would it require that abstinence be the treatment of choice in all cases.

Tenet 2: Abstinence is required because drinking of even moderate amounts of alcohol leads to a complete loss of control over alcohol consumption

'Alcoholism is a disease which manifests itself chiefly by the uncontrollable drinking of the victim'; '. . . an alcoholic cannot regain loss of control, even after years of abstinence the "compulsion" sets in on resumption of drinking'.[8] In other words, 'One drink, one drunk' (anonymous).

The idea that some people exhibit complete loss of control over the amount that they drink is the cornerstone of the abstinence position, and it is on this belief and not in the existence of a biochemical derangement (none has been discovered) exclusive to alcoholics that the recommendations of supporters of this position rest. Jellinek in his seminal work stated his proposal of a physiological disorder in the form of an hypothesis: 'I repeat that I regard the above merely as a working hypothesis but one which can be tested by means of the newer techniques in pharmacology, physiopathy and biochemistry'.[9] First, these 'newer techniques' have produced no evidence for a physiochemical disorder which is responsible for alcohol abuse. Second, the evidence flatly contradicts the strong form of the loss of control argument. Some critics give Jellinek the benefit of the doubt as to what he 'really' meant on this matter. (Jellinek is now dead, but his influence remains powerful.) While he may have offered scholarly reservations here and there in his writings, they appear to have played a small part in his general position. What *are* remembered, and are cited over and over again, are statements like the following: 'Loss of control [is used] to denote that stage in the development of their drinking history when the ingestion of *one* alcoholic drink sets up a *chain reaction* so that they are unable to adhere to their intention to "have one or two drinks only" but continue to ingest more and more—often with quite some difficulty and disgust—contrary to their volition'.

We have been at pains to refer to the disease-abstinence model, rather than just the disease model, as it is more commonly known, for it is on the loss-of-control hypothesis that clinical practice is shaped. Problem drinkers who approach clinics for assistance are routinely required to pledge abstinence, even though there is now sufficient evidence that for some better results are likely when controlled drinking is selected as the goal. (Assuredly *some* drinkers must be counselled to attempt abstinence, but others are likely to give up abusive drinking *only* when taught the cognitive and behavioural skills of controlled drinking, see Chapter 10.)

Rigid adherence to these two tenets leads to all problem drinkers being considered alcoholics and all alcoholics being made to agree to a lifetime of abstinence. In a recent study a number of people presented at clinics voicing concern about their use of alcohol. No one in the clinics was told that none had any alcohol problem; all were 'pseudopatients' who were careful not to behave as though they had any degree of alcohol dependence ('addiction'). The pseudopatients told the clinicians that they had come to the clinics for professional assessment of their problems. 'In the opinion of the investigators these agencies were particularly aggressive in selling their services. Of 29 assessments that were obtained, 17 indicated that the confederate [of the investigators] was an alcoholic; of these 17 cases, inpatient treatment was recommended nine times. The cost of the recommended treatments ranged from about US$6000 to $10 000 each, not including physicians' fees.' The majority of these individuals, not one of whom had an alcohol problem, were labelled 'alcoholic', and drastic steps, including hospitalisation, were promoted without reservation.[10]

In the interest of balance it should be said that the disease concept with all of its shortcominings is preferable to the moral condemnation meted out to inebriates in earlier years. But the treatment ideas and ideology of the disease-abstinence model lead to serious limitations in thinking about problem drinking and are leading to serious mistakes in the delivery of treatment services. An evaluation is overdue, and it must begin with the loss-of-control theory.

Strictly speaking the evaluation began over 20 years ago in the arguments of the early behaviour therapists. However, these environmentalists put their case in a strident way with ideology rather than facts to the fore and their views made little impact. The loss-of-control hypothesis is today accepted by most clinicians as long-since proved. The facts are that once alcohol is consumed, loss of control is not automatically triggered. Thus, traditional attitudes about what are and what are not acceptable treatment practices must be modified. There are two lines of evidence which have rendered the loss-of-control theory indefensible.

Priming studies

The theory holds that once alcohol enters the bloodstream it detonates a psychological 'craving' and complete loss of restraint over the intake of alcohol. A number of studies have been conducted to put these ideas to the test, and not one supports the craving/loss-of-control prediction. An early and most ingenious investigation was conducted in Alan Marlatt's laboratory at the University of Washington. He and his co-workers, Demming and Reid, recognised a serious methodological problem confronting researchers who seek an answer to the simple question: 'What happens to the psychological state of people who know that they are being given alcohol to drink?' If they do, in fact, report an increase in desire to drink following the administration of an alcoholic substance, is it because of the pharmacological effects of alcohol, or is it because they know that they have been given alcohol to drink? Cultural expectancies about the effects of alcohol can be likened to the ubiquitous placebo effects which have plagued medical researchers for decades. These were first noticed in therapies for people in pain. Patients may obtain relief from tablets labelled pain killers, even though they contain innocuous, pharmacologically inert substances. Somehow, in some people, the expectancy of relief leads to a real reduction in pain. Similarly, people given alcohol may have acquired certain culturally conditioned expectancies about the way people react to alcohol (i.e. become boisterous, uninhibited, drink in an unrestrained fashion, and so on). In saying this we are not saying that they are feigned responses. In research of this sort the difficulty is to separate the pharmacological from the cognitive effects of taking alcohol. Marlatt's solution to dissociate the two was elegant and simple.[11] Half the volunteers were given vodka in tonic (to disguise the taste) and the other half were given tonic alone. To complete the design, half each group was deceived as to the true content of the drink. Of those actually given vodka in their tonic, half were told that they were in the tonic-only group; half the tonic drinkers were led to believe that there was vodka in their drink. Figure 2.1 illustrates the conditions:

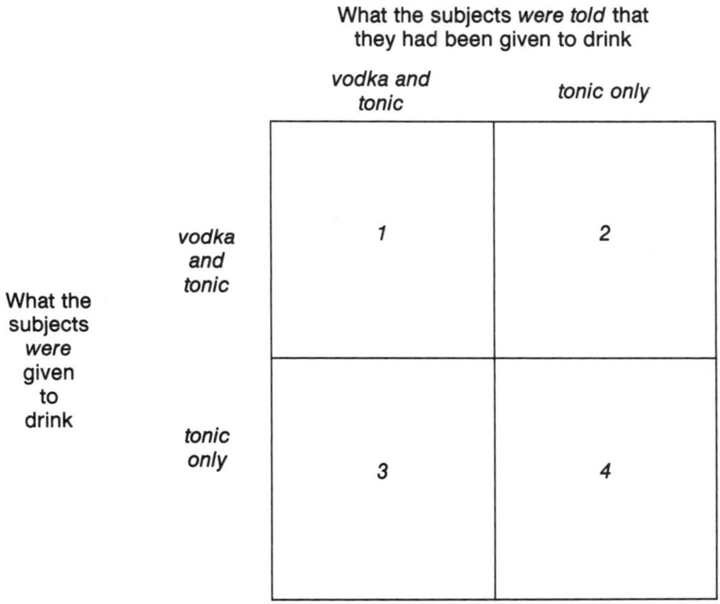

Figure 2.1 Design of Marlatt et al's loss of control drinking experiment

Marlatt gave subseqent drinking tests with the aim of separating and comparing the influence of the content of the instructions with the actual content of the drink on the behaviour of the volunteers. If the physiological effects of alcohol made the main difference, then groups 1 and 2 should have consumed the most in the tests, but if cognitions (expectancies, attitudes and beliefs) were of over-riding importance then those told that they had been given vodka in their tonic should have consumed more, regardless of whether they had been given vodka or not. The outcome was exactly in line with Marlatt's predictions: groups 1 and 3 taken together drank significantly more than groups 2 and 4, indicating that the drinkers' beliefs and expectancies were a more potent source of influence than the alcohol ingested.

Though the results seem to contradict the loss-on-control axiom, they are open to criticism. The volunteer subjects in the study were classified as moderate to heavy 'social drinkers'. Defenders of the abstinence position could deny the relevance of these results to the loss-of-control question because the subjects in the study were not alcoholics. In the absence of any criteria for deciding just who is and who is not an alcoholic, such a defence is irrefutable.

Priming studies with hospitalised alcoholics are not as easily dismissed. In these, and there are a number reviewed by Heather and Robertson,[12] individuals judged by medical personnel and the patients' own estimates to be suffering from alcohol problems were given surreptitious priming doses of alcohol. To name one study, Merry [13] supplied his patients with an ounce of vodka mixed in a large glass of orange juice. The mixture was described as a vitamin drink. After the patients had swallowed the drink they were assessed on tests designed to measure 'desire to drink'. These revealed no craving reactions or loss-of-control tendencies.

An interesting instance of controlled drinking in self-confessed alcoholics was 'controlled drinking' by clergymen members of abstinence groups who partook of communion wine in their daily services without lapsing into alcoholic binges.[14]

None of these results support the existence of a triggered process by which alcohol, once consumed, sets loose uncontrollable urges and paves the way for riotous drinking. To the contrary, the roles of context, dependency and expectancy are shown to be powerful determinants of 'craving' and drinking patterns.

Giving alcohol to chronic 'Skid Row' alcoholics over an extended period of time

There are a number of reports of studies of the behaviour of chronic 'Skid Row' drinkers who (a) volunteered to take part in studies, (b) did not want to be cured of their alcoholism (as they defined it), and (c) took part in the studies for monetary and other rewards. As participants, they were allowed to drink whisky, but only if they 'worked' for it (for example, by pressing a lever a number of times in order to get a shot of whisky). Others could drink beyond a certain level but if they did so they would have to forfeit certain privileges. In short, drinking was allowed up to very high levels, but external costs were applied when stipulated levels were exceeded. The findings from all these investigations agree that by the systematic manipulation of incentives and sanctions drinking can be increased or decreased. If the drinkers had to press the level on a 'rich' schedule of payoffs, they did so consistently. But when the demands were increased and the schedules made 'leaner', requiring more work per drink, the drinkers decided against continuing, even though had they chosen to continue working on the more demanding schedule they would have been able to collect their whisky reward.[15]

The important conclusions to come from these studies are:

1. The alcoholics did not drink at every opportunity. Instead, they initiated and terminated drinking episodes for reasons other than the availability and/or prior consumption of alcohol.
2. The subjects did not consume every drop of alcohol as soon as it became available. The majority consumed the alcohol they earned to drink later, at a time and place of their own choosing.
3. Even though some of the subjects showed clear signs of withdrawal reactions, such as hand tremors, they demonstrated a preference to 'save up' the alcohol they were receiving. Loss-of-control arguments would predict an even more dramatic loss of control in the face of withdrawal reactions, but this did not occur.
4. Some of the subjects tapered off their intake of alcohol so as to minimise the withdrawal reactions that would be likely if they drank at high and constant levels until the end of the experiment, when there would be no more whisky. All the evidence showed that these 'hopeless drunks' could engage in careful planning about the future and would forego some of the available alcohol in order to meet these plans.

These studies strike at the heart of conventional notions of loss of control and craving. To behavioural-environmental clinicians these results are not surprising. Why should not drinking, like any other behaviour, be subject to the laws of learning? And if a problem drinker's drinking is subject to these laws, then moderate drinking becomes a possibility.

This theoretical possibility has to be translated into practical, explicit guidelines, so that the clinician can obtain a reasonably good idea of who can and who cannot benefit from controlled drinking treatments. This is the subject of Chapter 3.

CHAPTER 3

Controlled Drinking, Abstinence and Dependency

In Chapter 2 the evidence against the disease-abstinence position was reviewed. Its major theoretical drawback is that treatments derived from it emphasise the existence of a physical disorder located within particular individuals called alcoholics, while external influences are accorded little significance in aetiology and treatment. In principle, therapy for these 'sick' individuals proceeds through three stages:

1. Medical detoxification where necessary;
2. Lectures to the patient on the fundamental and ineradicable defect of alcoholism—an irreversible disorder which will always leave him powerless to control his alcohol intake once drinking begins; and
3. Clinical intervention designed to elicit from the patient an admission that he is an alcoholic and, ideally, a statement of willingness to join an abstinence society (for example, Alcoholics Anonymous, Syanon) of similarly afflicted individuals.

This, in schematic outline, is the conceptual framework of the disease-abstinence model. If there are no exceptions to this formula, it is also true that commonsense never left the day-to-day work of medical/disease-abstinence practitioners. Only the strawman clinician of behaviourist imagination ignored altogether the coexistant difficulties in the drinker's life and their role in his unhappiness. In our experience, those who work within the medical model are capable of shrewd insights into the self-defeating habits of the drinker's lifestyle and the significance of interpersonal relationships. However, it is fair to say that there has been no place in their theory for a systematic analysis of the social-environmental influences that contribute to the onset and maintenance of problem drinking. Furthermore, to them the idea of certain drinkers themselves learning to assess and master these influences as a prelude to the establishment of moderate drinking goals is an anathema.

The behaviourists in the 1960s and 1970s, when they discussed alcoholism, displayed an untroubled optimism on this very point. ('Alcoholism' was a word they avoided wherever possible, only using it to indicate an area of study.) Controlled drinking was not merely a theoretical possibility but, perhaps with a few exceptions, a reality within reach of all problem drinkers. Their starting point was a belief that the causes of excessive drinking lay in the drinker's environment—causes that they insisted were fully understood, as indeed, it was assumed, were the causes of all behaviour. One of the most popular advanced textbooks on behaviour modification exemplifies this view. It has no listing in its index for 'alcoholism', 'drinking problems', 'agoraphobia', 'schizophrenia', 'depression' or 'sleeping disorders', to name a few of the more surprising omissions. The reason for the omissions is not difficult to find. If the laws of conditioning and learning can fully account for the development of all behaviour, be it 'normal' or 'abnormal', then clearly the correct application of rewards and punishments will modify behaviour in whatever direction is desired. This simplistic approach gave way in the late 1970s and 1980s to a more sophisticated interpretation of psychological disorders. Skinnerian and classical conditioning influences were retained within an expanded and more complex system which gave primary importance to cognitive (mental) influences. After 50 years, thinking and feeling had returned to psychology. But, as with the 'basic laws of conditioning', the explanatory staple of the earlier mechanistic accounts of behaviour, the 'laws' of cognition (thinking) and affect (emotion) were also framed in general terms assumed to apply in the same way to all behavioural and psychological problems. Thus the search for systematic individual differences was also given little attention by cognitive-behavioural clinicians. The assumption that alcoholics (problem drinkers in their terminology) make up a homogeneous group was accepted from the outset.

Drinking problems were conceptualised not as collections of physiological dysfunctions but instead as behavioural excesses, differing only in degree from one patient to the next and modifiable in a downward direction.[1] As a group the cognitive-behavioural writers tend to be forceful advocates of controlled drinking, the techniques of which are discussed in detail later in the book. The two chief objections voiced against controlled drinking are openly acknowledged and answered in behavioural writings, save for the crucial homogeneity flaw, which is at the centre of most current battles between the two models. The two objections and the behaviourists' replies to them are as follows:

Objection: As the old saying has it, 'if it is not broken, don't fix it'. Since Alcoholics Anonymous and other abstinence approaches do *work, why then experiment with something that may not do as well?*

Reply: *Does* abstinence therapy, in any of its forms, work? A close examination of the clinical evidence does not tell an optimistic story. There are no outcome figures published by AA, but the available literature indicates a drop-out rate of up to 80 per cent, or higher.[2] Claims of 50 per cent success have been made, but that number is 50 per cent of the 10 to 20 per cent who remain as regular attenders, giving a success rate of 5 to 10 per cent. Baekeland[3] puts it at no higher than 25 per cent, still a very discouraging figure. While these data are not an indictment of AA, they do question the belief that, to be 'cured', the drinker must take the pledge of abstinence. Similar and equally discouraging improvement rates were noted in the US Government sponsored Rand Report. The authors of the report followed up patients treated at hundreds of Alcohol Treatment Centers across the United States, at which abstinence was the only goal discussed. The results showed that only 28 per cent of the patients had remained sober for six months, and this figure dropped to 7 per cent at four-year follow-up. For serious problem drinkers in some categories (for example, younger, unmarried patients) success rates were higher if the patients opted for controlled drinking, for which they were given no support or training. To the findings of the Rand Report we can add the overview of 80 similar studies compiled by Costello et al.[4] The average success rate achieved ('abstinent' plus those 'still drinking but improved') was 26 per cent or slightly lower.

The best success rate, therefore, that can be claimed for abstinence-oriented treatments is 25 per cent, and the true figure is probably much lower. These figures require that alternative methods of treatment be explored.

Objection: Why should alcoholics be encouraged to try controlled drinking when so many have tried and failed?

Reply: This objection, though debateable because of its sweeping conclusions, is one which cannot be dismissed out of hand. In a 1985 article in the prestigious *New England Journal of Medicine,* Helzer et al. reviewed the clinical outcomes of 1289 patients assessed over a 10 year period.[5] The assessment methods were rigorous and the follow-up efforts were a model of persistence. The number of patients who were able to satisfy the investigators that they were drinking in a moderate fashion made up less than 5 per cent of the original sample. On the basis of these results Helzer and his colleagues questioned the wisdom of offering controlled drinking programmes to any alcoholics seeking treatment. Twenty years earlier Fox[6] also expressed serious reservations about moderate drinking: 'Among my own approximately 3000 patients not one has been able to achieve moderation although every one of them has tried'.

These claims cannot be ignored, but some caution must be exercised in taking the arguments, if not the data, at face value. For one thing, there is the vicious circularity which has been used on more than one occasion. It is an after-the-fact argument, which goes something like this. Once the results are in, the question is asked: 'Did the patient learn and maintain controlled drinking?' If the answer is in the affirmative then the response is: 'Well, then he could not have been a true alcoholic, could he?' The next question is: 'And the other patient, how did he fare on follow-up examination?' To the answer that he is still drinking heavily, the response comes: 'Well, that patient was a true alcoholic'. The case is considered proved but nothing is learned.

Another reservation is that none of Helzer's clinicians took any steps to equip the patient with the skills necessary to achieve the status of long-term moderate drinker. On this point Miller's criticisms are well taken: 'These [moderate drinking outcomes in former alcoholics] have been, for the most part, incidental moderation outcomes because patients have been provided with no assistance or encouragement toward moderation. If anything they have been told that moderation efforts are doomed to ultimate failure'.[7] We know of cases where well-intentioned practitioners have forecast personality disintegration and even death if ever the patient attempted controlled drinking. As Miller says: 'It is hardly surprising that such patients often fail to achieve moderation; no more surprising than the failure of obese patients to lose weight when told to do so but given no encouragement, guidance or reinforcement in that effort'.[8] More than that, 'failure' is virtually mandated when patients are counselled in dramatic terms that to have one more drink is tantamount to coming to the edge of a full-blown relapse. It is difficult to conceive of a strategy more conducive to what Marlatt refers to as the abstinence violation effect. Patients are forcibly told that their behaviour with regard to alcohol can be categorised in but one of two ways: total success (complete abstinence) or total failure (having a single drink). If they do lapse and have a few drinks they can be vulnerable to acts of catastrophic self-labelling: 'I've gone back to square one, the treatment has been a total failure, what's the use—I've failed . . . May as well have another and another.'

Abstinence treatments have a dismal record and controlled drinking programmes can hardly be expected to constitute an improvement if they are denigrated and then ignored. The acid test is the outcome of treatments where controlled drinking is endorsed and taught from the outset. Until the mid-1980s the record of controlled drinking treatments was encouraging and seemed to confirm the optimism of its adherents. The picture is now less clear and the vituperative arguments, million dollar lawsuits and challenges to the veracity and integrity of some of the key investigators has thrown the field into confusion. A disinterested review of the main experiments is needed to clear it up. The successes and, even more, the failures, can provide the basis for an integrated position and the development of specific guidelines which can tell us when to recommend and when to advise against controlled drinking.

Controlled drinking: an evaluation and new directions

The first shots in the battle between the proponents of abstinence and those who supported controlled drinking were fired following the appearance in 1962 of a paper by D.L. Davies in the *Quarterly Journal of Studies on Alcohol*.[9] The cause of the furor was the publication of evidence for 'normal drinking by recovered alcohol addicts' in seven of 93 patients that he followed for periods between seven and 11 years. Davies himself was no propagandist for controlled drinking and he presented his findings simply because he thought they could be of some interest. To his dismay the paper unleashed a storm of critical protest, most of it directed against him. He was personally censured and a special supplement to an issue of the *Quarterly Journal* was published in which he was virtually accused of heresy. Worse yet, those who funded Davies' research attempted to persuade him to leave out any mention of these 'embarrassing' findings in his report. To his credit, Davies resisted them.

The harsh antagonisms between abstinence and controlled drinking clinicians live on and the 'paradigm clash' is far from settled. When, in 1982, the *Journal of Studies on Alcohol* published a number of articles with conclusions similar to those published by the Rand Corporation[10] one major contributor to alcoholism research proceeded to cut the Rutger's Centre of Alcohol Studies, the journal's publisher, out of his will.

The next chapter in the story was written with the publication of the aforementioned Rand Report. It, too, found evidence of long-term (four year) controlled drinking in ex-patients from clinics where, as remarked earlier, no clinical assistance was given in the acquisition of controlled drinking. The response of the alcohol establishment was, and still is, extremely hostile to those who take up this work. Here is a sample of this hostility from T.G. Terbell, chairman of the board of the National Council on Alcoholism: 'Abstinence from alcohol is necessary for recovery from the disease of alcoholism'. And about studies demonstrating controlled drinking: 'There is a need for *responsible* research, carried out with proper controls as well as the *judicious* publication of results where pertinent' (emphasis added). Given his pronouncedly threatening tone it is difficult to avoid concluding that the powerful NCA intends to discourage researchers from pursuing certain 'heresies' and, where necesssary, to use their influence to block the publication of research that they do not deem 'responsible'. Their sympathisers in the US Congress have stated that the government body responsible for funding research into alcohol studies, the National Institute on Alcohol Abuse and Alcoholism, 'will want to reevaluate ... grants for scientific research to see that there is not a repeat of this type of damage' that is, it will stop the funding of any more reports that might produce findings like those of the Rand Report.

Putting aside attack and invective, one valid reservation about the Davies[11] report, Kendall and Stanton's[12] on the resumption of moderate drinking by untreated drinkers, and the data from the thousands of patients surveyed in the Rand Report, is that none of these reports contained scientific controls. All refer to 'incidental' adjustments to controlled drinking in those treated by clinical personnel emphasising abstinence as the only safe cure for excessive drinking.

This criticism does not apply to the famous Lovibond and Caddy Australian investigation which set out to prove the viability of moderate drinking in a group of individuals with long histories of alcohol abuse.[13] Lovibond and Caddy employed a rigorous methodology and thorough follow-up assessments, and found that 85 per cent of their subjects improved significantly when tested at post-therapy intervals ranging from four months to more than a year. At the two-year follow-up assessment an impressive 59 per cent of the subjects treated with behavioural techniques were still drinking in a controlled manner.

But still the issue remained unsettled. Those favouring the abstinence-disease position could concede the validity of the Lovibond and Caddy data and yet voice the same old objections. 'Yes, these people were excessive drinkers, and they did change from excessive to controlled drinking, but they were not *real* alcoholics.'

In an effort to settle the question once and for all the Sobells[14] embarked on an ambitious programme to teach controlled drinking to patients diagnosed as 'true' alcoholics by orthodox clinicians working at Patton State Hospital in California. One group was given Individualised Behaviour Therapy (IBT) for controlled drinking and another received the care routinely given to diagnosed alcoholics to bring about abstinence. IBT was the name of a package of behavioural self-control treatments (including counselling, aversive components, problem solving and assertiveness training). A group of 70 males, all of whom were diagnosed as severe (gamma) alcoholics and who had admitted themselves to Patton State Hospital for treatment, were randomly assigned to the different conditions. All the volunteers had had at least one previous episode of hospitalisation for alcohol problems. The programme lasted for four weeks. At the end of treatment, and at two-year follow-up, those who were trained in IBT to drink in a controlled fashion achieved a much better adjustment after release from the hospital than those in the other major treatment group. The Sobells' study was a landmark investigation. First, no one disputed the 'alcoholic' status of the volunteers. Second, whatever the label given to the hospitalised patients, all exhibited alcohol problems considerably more severe than those of the Lovibond and Caddy volunteers. Third, because no other study of the long-term efficacy of treatment for alcoholism—behavioural or non-behavioural—has followed so many patients for such an extended period of time the Sobells' study is of particular significance, especially since follow-up contracts were conducted at least once a month over this long period (over the phone, by one of the Sobells).

The impact of the Sobells work was felt worldwide. It seemed that the question was settled: controlled drinking taught via behavioural techniques was a possibility for *all* drinkers. A corollary was that all that distinguished 'alcoholics' from 'excessive drinkers' were the labels themselves. Defenders of the environmental position rushed to the conclusion that excessive drinking (alcoholism/problem drinking) was the result of habit and upbringing and was not an incurable physical disorder.

So it stood until 1982 when Pendery, Maltzman and West[15] published a report in *Science* challenging the findings in the Sobells' study. Pendery and her colleagues announced that a 10-year follow-up investigation of the patients treated by the Sobells revealed that only one of the 20 patients in the IBT controlled drinking group could be rated as a non-problem drinker. They presented evidence which, if correct, documented severe and early relapses, in one case within eight days of discharge from the IBT programme. Of the 20 in the IBT group, six have since died, four from alcohol-related disabilities. The Pendery et al. paper contained medical records of the rehospitalisation of the IBT patients, which occurred in some cases within weeks of discharge. Subject 4: 'Readmitted to Patton 8 days after discharge ... left Patton State Hospital 8 days ago, resumed drinking the next day and now earnestly requests Voluntary Alcoholic readmission. He is tremulous ... is now actively hallucinating, feels he may go into DTs.' And from the record of another, Subject 8: 'Readmitted to Patton 13 days after his discharge ... this ... intoxicated man is taken in on 72 hour hold, partly because he is suicidal . . . This patient was admitted . . . so intoxicated he did not even recall his own name.' Subject 7, readmitted to Patton three months, 22 days after discharge: 'Requests admission for treatment of alcoholism—was here previously . . . he thinks he might be close to DTs as he feels confused, sees pictures flash before his eyes and sees little moving objects on the floor . . . he is grossly tremulous.' The records of these and other patients in the controlled drinking group led Pendery et al. to describe the treatment as an unqualified failure.

In their defence the Sobells published a rebuttal in 1984 in a paper entitled 'The Aftermath of a Heresy'. In it they criticised Pendery et al. for failing to note that, badly as the controlled drinking experimental group performed, the patients treated along traditional lines fared significantly worse. Moreover, the controlled drinking subjects did better in the second year after treatment. These are valid counter-arguments, but allowing for them the results still suggest that drinkers of this severity are not good prospects for controlled drinking (or any treatment, judging from the even more depressing results from the patients given traditional treatment).

The Dickens Committee, a committee of prestigious scientific and legal professionals, was convened in Canada to investigate the personal integrity of the Sobells, which had been questioned, along with their results. The committee found no reasonable cause to doubt either. But a vexing question remains: can those with severe drinking problems ever return to social drinking? From Helzer et al. in 1985[16] we are told: 'The evolution to stable moderate drinking appears to be a rare outcome among alcoholics treated at medical or psychiatric facilities . . . If moderate drinking is an exceedingly rare outcome we may do a serious disservice to the majority of . . . patients by implying a professional sanction of attempts to drink moderately.' Against this is the conclusion arrived at by Miller in his 1983 review of a large literature on the success of controlled drinking: 'moderation-oriented approaches hold at least as much promise as abstinence-oriented methods *in treating less dependent problem drinkers*' (emphasis added).

These italicised words suggest a resolution of the contrasting findings, which is to distinguish low from high dependent drinkers. This is an obvious challenge to the homogeneity assumption that all alcoholics/problem drinkers share a common biochemical flaw or faulty upbringing (depending on one's theoretical preference). If the homogeneity assumption is true, then when confronting the Rand Report, Lovibond, Helzer, Sobell, Miller et al.'s cacophony of results, all that can be said of controlled drinking is that some can manage it and others cannot. The problem, of course, is to predict who will be able to and who will not. To put it another way, we must ask: 'Are there individual differences which distinguish those drinkers with a good prognosis for controlled drinking, for abstinence or for any improvement at all?'

From the earliest writings on alcoholism, writers have speculated on individual personality differences and their connection to drinking (see below), but the only categorisation based on the drinker's actual reactions to alcohol (as opposed to hypothesised personality disorders) that has gained any following was put together by Jellinek.[17] He proposed the existence of at least five species or categories of alcoholism. The logic of his scheme is founded on the premise that the differences between the varieties were qualitative and not just ones of degree. The five are:

Alpha alcoholism This term referred to people with a purely psychological dependence on alcohol. Jellinek called alpha alcoholics those who display neither loss of control nor the inability to abstain. They use alcohol to assuage emotional distress and to help them combat the stresses in their lives. This misuse of alcohol may lead to work or family problems, but Jellinek felt that a progression from alpha to the other forms of alcoholism was not inevitable. Alpha alcoholics, he noted, were often called 'problem drinkers' by other writers.

Beta alcoholism Jellinek reserved this category for those who suffer physical damage (cirrhosis, gastritis) resulting from excessive drinking, but no psychological or physiological dependence. Beta alcoholism is likely to be encountered in groups or societies where heavy drinking is combined with an inadequate diet.

Gamma alcoholism This category is closest to the popular conceptions of the alcoholic. Jellinek listed, amongst other characteristics of gamma alcoholics: large changes in tolerance (i.e. needing progressively more alcohol to achieve the same effect); withdrawal reactions (physical and psychological distress reactions after a period of abstinence); and loss of control over drinking. He speculated that there is an inexorable progression from psychological to physical dependence (a state of need which, if not satisfied, leads to aversive withdrawal reactions). Jellinek defined gamma alcoholism as the most devastating variety, whether measured in terms of physical destruction or social dislocation. He wrote that gamma alcoholics passed through four distinct stages in their drinking:

(a) *Prealcoholic* At the start though the individual may not differ outwardly from 'normal' drinkers, alcohol becomes the standard means of handling stressful situations. The prealcoholic phase could last from a few months to two years or more.

(b) *Prodromal* (meaning a warning or signalling of a disease) Jellinek said that this phase begins suddenly. The crucial indicators are 'alcoholic palimpsets' or blackouts. Blackout when used in this sense means amnesia about some or all aspects of a drinking bout; an inability to recall events when sobriety returns ('Did I do that?'). In the prodromal stage the alcoholic begins to 'sneak' drinks before social gatherings, and gulps drinks at other times. By this time the person will have acquired the reputation of a 'hard drinker' but may excite no suspicions in those around him about the growing disorder. Jellinek listed the time span of the prodromal period as between six months and five years.

(c) *Crucial* This is the third phase of gamma alcoholism. The main index is loss of control over drinking. On reaching this stage, whenever the person takes a drink a chain reaction is set in motion. It is within the person's power to decide whether or not to begin drinking, but after beginning he is powerless to regulate his intake. The difficulties with alcohol are now apparent to those close to him. The drinker becomes aware of the need for rationalisations and at the same time begins a series of ultimately futile attempts to regain control. As these efforts invariably fail, his response to drinking is to alternate between foolish optimism and an angry, despairing remorse. Alcohol becomes the major preoccupation of his life and obtaining and maintaining a supply of liquor takes precedence over all other recreations and responsibilities. Serious troubles make their appearance in his family life, occupational activities and friendships. It is around this time, if not before, that alcohol-linked hospitalisations become necessary (for example, for injuries sustained in falls when intoxicated).

(d) *Chronic* Jellinek postulates this as the fourth and final phase of gamma alcoholism. Some drinkers in the third, crucial, phase may be able to hold onto a job and keep their social relationships more or less intact, but in the chronic phase morning drinking becomes a common occurrence, serving to relieve intense withdrawal reactions. Intoxication becomes a daily event and a process of downward social drift begins. The company of other heavy drinkers is sought and the gamma alcoholic finds himself losing competence and control in every area of his life. Serious and obvious physical changes take place in the drinker and severe psychiatric disorders, growing all the while, become incapacitating. If the gamma alcoholic does not maintain a balanced diet, brain damage will result.

Delta alcoholism This variety resembles gamma alcoholism, with physical and psychological dependence being present. The main difference between them is that delta alcoholics do not suffer loss of control once they begin drinking. However, they cannot refrain from drinking for more than a day or two, at most, without suffering withdrawal symptoms.

Epsilon alcoholism Jellinek had little to say about this category except to speculate that these were the episodic or 'binge' drinkers who did not exhibit physical dependence on alcohol.

While outlining these five types of alcoholism, Jellinek did not deny the possibility of still other categories. He classified only the gamma and delta varieties as diseases, and was open in his thinking as to their origin: 'Learning theory . . . does not exclude any other etiological theories; it can be complimentary to any of them. Neither would it conflict with a disease conception of one or the other species of alcoholism.'[18]

The careful descriptive work of Jellinek outlining the typical train of symptoms exhibited by the most disturbed drinkers has been of great value to clinicians and theoreticians. He broke with orthodox thinking which recognised only two classes of drinkers—'normal' (light or heavy) and 'alcoholic'. But for all these advances, Jellinek's categorisations are static, still retain the loss-of-control notions (in the gamma and delta species), and are couched in disease model terminology. His commitment to the disease-abstinence position ignores situational, cultural and cognitive influences on drinking behaviour. Furthermore, diagnostic reliabilities for distinguishing one brand of alcoholism from another are far too low to be acceptable. The benefits of Jellinek's thinking to the field of alcohol studies today is the wealth of descriptive detail he provided and the emphasis on the concept of dependence which, in the hands of Edwards, Gross, Hodgson and their group, have helped to resolve the contradictions which appeared to indicate that controlled drinking programmes were sometimes better and sometimes worse than abstinence therapies.

Notions of dependence in theory and clinical practice

In his five-fold classification scheme, Jellinek focussed most of his attention on the drinkers labelled as gamma alcoholics. He claimed that they were the only ones to lose control after starting to drink. They also exhibit signs of tolerance, suffer withdrawal symptoms and are dependent both psychologically and physically on alcohol. No defence seems possible for the strong form of the loss-of-control hypothesis, and the weak after-the-fact form is infinitely flexible and thus useless, but the ideas of tolerance, withdrawal and dependence are valuable.

Tolerance refers to the changes in response to alcohol with repeated and regular exposure to it. There is a slight metabolic tolerance, which allows the body to process alcohol (metabolise it) more efficiently. In parallel there are pronounced increases in behavioural and psychological tolerance which mean that with regular, heavy drinking the amounts of alcohol needed to cause gross mental and behavioural intoxication increases. (It is worth adding here, though we will come to it later, that the experienced excessive drinker's tolerance is in well learned/highly practiced responses like simple conversation; more subtle tests for problem-solving and skill-learning will reveal impairments even though the drinker shows no gross deficits in simple or well-learned responses.) With steady drinking the individual 'gets used to it' and requires more alcohol to produce the same effects. Tolerance is a sign of the nervous system's ability to adapt to alcohol. As far as is known, this occurs in all people and is a function of a person's drinking history—the heavier a person's drinking, the higher his tolerance. (A full account of tolerance is given in Chapter 8.)

Withdrawal refers to a set of reactions shown by chronic drinkers when they go without alcohol. It appears following the development of high levels of tolerance, though not all people with high levels of tolerance experience withdrawal reactions. Those with withdrawal reactions are said to exhibit dependence, but the two phenomena are best considered as separate but interrelated reactions to excessive drinking. There is no agreed-upon list of dependence reactions, but the following, described by Griffith Edwards,[19] the leading writer on the topic, are found on most lists:

(a) *Narrowing of the drinking repertoire* Unlike the ordinary drinker, whose place of drinking, intake and choice of drink will vary from time to time, the dependent individual will drink on a rigid schedule and, when possible, the same type of drink. 'The syndrome must be pictured as subtle and plastic rather than as something set hard, but as dependence advances the pattern tends to become increasingly hardened'.[20]

(b) *Salience of drinking* As dependence increases the drinker begins to disregard his obligations and non-drinking activities in which he once took enjoyment. Less time is spent with children, and friends who drink moderately, and thoughts of how and when to procure alcohol become the most vital considerations in his life.

(c) *Tolerance* While this has been mentioned above, one point worth repeating is the loose coupling between tolerance and dependence: 'The rate of development of tolerance is variable, but the heavy drinker who is not dependent can manifest considerable tolerance'.[21] In later stages of dependence the drinker may 'lose' his tolerance and become badly intoxicated by amounts of alcohol he once handled without obvious difficulty. Tolerance to alcohol can extend to other drugs (for example, minor tranquillisers). Since polydrug use is increasingly common, the clinician should make the patient aware of the potential for serious problems if alcohol is taken along with other drugs.

(d) *Withdrawal symptoms* In the early stages withdrawal reactions are not severe and may be intermittent. They will not incapacitate the drinker and some of the reactions listed below may appear alone or with just a few others. With high dependence, however, the drinker will experience an array of withdrawal reactions which typically have their onset in the morning just after waking, though they may occur at other times when the alcohol level in the body falls sharply. Withdrawal reactions require heavy drinking (for example, a bottle of spirits per day or its equivalent for a few years), but the time to first onset will vary from one person to the next. The reactions include tremor ('the shakes') which affect the hands or even the whole body; morning nausea, which may lead the drinker to avoid food; sweating during the night, which may be so copious that the drinker wakes from his sleep soaking wet; and mood disturbances, which in milder forms can manifest as 'edginess'. The more severe variety presents as extreme agitation and depression, combined with an exceptional sensitivity to noises bordering on strong fright reactions. Along with these, Edwards mentions 'impaired control', by which he means deciding not to exercise control, 'craving' for alcohol, and a sense of compulsion to drink which the drinker attempts, unsuccessfully, to resist.

The value of the dependence concept is that, unlike the label 'alcoholism', the components of dependence can be specified, measured and experimentally investigated. The predictive value of dependence has been demonstrated in laboratory experiments and suggests a resolution for the otherwise puzzling contradictions wherein some studies demonstrate and others deny the possibility of controlled drinking.

In a study run along the lines of the Marlatt, Demming and Reid experiment described in the previous chapter, the English workers Hodgson, Stockwell and Rankin gave a group of hospitalised drinkers vodka or juice to drink. As in the Marlatt et al. experiment, half each group was deceived and the other half told the truth about the contents of their drink. The chief difference between the Marlatt experiment and this one was the measurement of dependence. Hodgson et al. gave all the patients the SADQ (Severity of Alcohol Dependence Questionnaire)[22] and on the basis of their results formed two groups, one made up of high and the other of low alcohol dependent patients. For those in the low dependence group, like Marlatt's subjects, the rate of drinking was influenced by what they believed they had been drinking. However, the opposite was true of the high dependence subjects; for them the contents of the drink rather than the content of the instructions determined the speed of drinking. The results demonstrated that severely dependent subjects were more disposed to drink 60 minutes after consuming alcohol in the juice than those in the juice only condition, regardless of whether they believed that the priming drinks contained alcohol. Cognitive factors assumed greater importance for the drinking behaviour of less dependent subjects.

In another study Skinner and Allen asked problem drinkers whether they thought they could cut down to 'a few drinks a day'. Of the patients who scored low levels of dependence (measured in this case by the Alcohol Dependence Scale, ADS) the majority answered in the affirmative. Those who scored at the high end of the ADS answered 'no' to the same question.[23]

Stockwell et al. administered the SADQ to 53 hospitalised patients who were undergoing withdrawal from alcohol. SADQ scores correlated significantly with the amount of medication given to ameliorate withdrawal reactions. That is, the higher the dependence scores, the more medication they received.

Skinner and Allen looked at the relationship between dependence (measured by the ADS) and 'thinking disorder, hypochondriasis, persecutory ideas, self-deprecation, anxiety, depression and impulsiveness'. They found highly significant relationships ($p<.05$ to $p<.001$) between ADS scores and these personality variables. This is an interesting and important finding in the light of the often mentioned claims that certain personality disorders stand in a causal relationship to alcoholism. The Skinner and Allen findings raise a different set of explanatory possibilities. One possibility is that personality disorders are correlated with, but not causal of, excessive drinking; another is that chronic levels of drinking lead to the combination of physical, psychological and social difficulties that are compressed into the expression 'personality disorders'.

For the clinician the payoff value of a concept lies in its contribution to predicting treatment outcome. Here, too, the measurement of dependence is of demonstrable value. Orford, Oppenheimer and Edwards[24] looked at the factors which distinguished, at two-year follow-up, drinkers who opted for abstinence from those who maintained controlled drinking. Not one of the controlled drinkers had been labelled a gamma alcoholic, while the majority of the abstainers had attracted a gamma classification. These results are only suggestive because measures of dependence were not taken and the reliability of the Jellinek system is not high. Nevertheless the quite reasonable assumption is that the gamma patients would have scored higher on the SADQ, the ADS or one of the other tests for dependence. On this line of reasoning, a further prediction is that problem drinkers (whatever their actual intake of alcohol) who score in the low range of dependence would be more likely to succeed at controlled drinking, while highly dependent drinkers would be risks for anything but complete abstinence. (Those in the middle range could negotiate the goal to be selected, according to past history of alcohol problems, and so on.)

This is exactly what Polich, Armor and Braiker[25] found in their examination of the Rand Report follow-up data. Their conclusions were complex but, boiled down to their essentials, they stated that the 'results were consistent with Edwards' emphasis on alcohol dependence, suggesting that the ability to maintain non-problem drinking decreases as the severity of dependence increases'. And the fact that the one person in the Sobells' group of 20 who was best able to carry on with controlled drinking was the drinker who showed the fewest signs of dependence is consistent with the propositions about the relationship between dependence levels and controlled drinking.

None of the foregoing should be taken to indicate that the low dependence excessive drinker is necessarily in better health than his highly dependent counterpart. Wodak, Saunders and their co-workers studied 193 patients with alcoholic liver disease. SADQ ratings were obtained and the findings are intriguing and worthy of consideration. Sixty-three per cent showed low dependence (SADQ scores <15), 20 per cent showed moderate dependence (SADQ 15–30) and 17 per cent were rated as severely dependent (SADQ >30). From these results the authors concluded that 'patients who escape florid symptoms of alcohol dependence are at greater risk of developing liver damage because they are able to sustain a continual consumption for many years'.[26]

Two more studies will complete our brief review. In an English study[27] 37 subjects who scored in the lower ranges of dependence were taught controlled drinking. Later, 61 per cent were categorised at follow-up assessment as 'successes+improved', a vastly higher figure than the 4 per cent reported in 1985 by Helzer et al. in the *New England Journal of Medicine*. Helzer's group did not give systematic data on dependence, but the speculation would be that their patients would have fallen into the high range. If correct, Helzer et al.'s conclusion that 'the evolution to stable moderate drinking appears to be a rare outcome among alcoholics' could be rewritten with more accuracy as 'the evolution to stable moderate drinking appears to be a rare outcome among highly dependent drinkers.' It could be added that heavy but low dependence drinkers do worse, if urged to adopt complete abstinence.

Sanchez-Craig and her colleagues randomly assigned 70 heavy (but low dependence) drinkers to identical cognitive-behavioural treatments. The main findings of the study are as follows: by the end of treatment the group which had the abstinence goal imposed upon them reduced their drinking by a significant amount, but were still drinking twice as much as the problem drinkers assigned to the controlled drinking goal. Sanchez-Craig commented: 'It was concluded that for most early stage problem drinkers [their drinking levels were not trivial, averaging out to about three bottles of spirits per week] a goal of moderation may be more suitable than a goal of abstinence. First, moderation was more acceptable for the majority of clients; second, clients in the moderate-drinking condition drank less during treatment; third, most of the clients who were assigned to abstinence developed moderate drinking on their own; and lastly, the clients in the abstinence group requested more aftercare appointments.'[28]

The concept of alcohol dependence is well grounded in empirical investigations and deserves to supplant the more popular diagnostic label 'alcoholic'. It does not carry the stigma of the latter; it allows for finer differentiations amongst the population of problem drinkers; it supplies a continuum along which all drinkers can be located; and, it has important implications for the answer to the crucial question in alcohol treatment: 'moderate drinking or total abstinence?'. Lastly, it helps to bring order to a collection of controversial studies and seemingly contradictory outcomes.

The continued interest in alcohol dependence is further strengthened by its recognition in the latest edition of the *Diagnostic and Statistical Manual (DSM III)* in which a distinction is made between 'alcohol abuse' and 'alcohol dependence'. As *DSM III* is the most authoritative diagnostic manual in the English-speaking world we can expect that these terms will soon filter into everyday use. However, the *DSM III* criteria are poorly specified, have unacceptably low reliabilities,[29] and alcohol dependence (303.9x) is treated as an all or nothing problem. In this form the entry can be of no more than heuristic value.

There is a debit side in the use of dependence as the explanation of drinking problems. To begin with there is the term 'dependence syndrome' which has achieved widespread usage. There is a real risk that this term will come to be accepted as a synonym for 'addict' or 'alcoholic' and thus will give backdoor entry to the notions of disease and loss of control. Edwards, the leader in this area, has been at pains to stress the interaction of biological, psychological and cultural factors in dependence specifically, and excessive drinking generally. However, as Sanchez-Craig remarks, it is the rule for those in the field of alcohol studies to ignore judicious warnings. Another limitation is that while many of the components of dependence have immediate face validity, obtaining precise and reliable definitions and measurements is an unfinished task. For example, 'increased salience of alcohol', to take one of the components mentioned by Edwards, or 'narrowing of the drinking repertoire', to take another, have an intuitive face value, but no one has yet developed reliable measures for them. Tremor, sweating and the physical indices of dependence present fewer problems, but there is still a great deal of work to do before there are adequate, operational definitions for the more subjective elements of the 'syndrome'.

The most serious mistake of all would be to present excessive drinking and alcohol-related problems as disorders whose causes, as before, are located 'within' the drinker but which are now called his 'dependence syndrome' instead of his alcoholism. Drinkers, whether of low, moderate or high dependence, have to contend with relationships, obligations and stressors in a real world. It is the interplay between these influences and the psychobiological processes of dependence which form the basis for comprehending alcohol problems and planning the strategies of therapy.

CHAPTER 4

Environmental Influences and Conventional Expectations About the Effects of Alcohol

Apart from the study of dependence, the second major development in the understanding of alcohol problems in recent years has come from a systematic study of the effects of environmental influences and the drinker's cognitions and beliefs that are habitually brought to bear on the situational emotional stressors he faces. This work has expanded the range of investigations enormously and with each finding the scope of therapeutic possibilities has increased proportionately. The thrust of this research is into the drinking behaviour itself and its immediate antecedents, and away from speculations about deep personality processes. Prior to the 1970s very little empirical work had been done into this most basic area of alcoholism. Mark Sobell commented, tongue a little in cheek, that drinking behaviour is, by definition, a fairly important part of drinking problems. Yet, when he and his colleagues set out to compile and review information on it they discovered that good data on the topic were virtually nonexistent. Those searching the literature could find statements of the sort that informed the reader that 'an alcoholic drinks in a manner so as to become drunk'.[1] Sobell remarked that although the import of such deductive logic did not escape them, it was hardly a sufficient foundation for constructing a useful account of how problem drinkers behave with alcohol, or the influences to which they respond.[2] Indeed, the general belief among alcohol specialists was that the drinking behaviour of 'alcoholics' was essentially invulnerable to the manipulation of environmental variables. Drinking was universally believed to be symptomatic of deeper and more significant problems (referred to variously as troubled souls, unconscious conflicts, personality disorders and physiochemical disorders). The world outside the drinker was of relatively little interest compared with the world within.

If that is so, it is hard to reconcile beliefs in inner causation with the commonplace observations that alcohol problems are consistently higher in some countries than others. Table 4.1 gives the per capita figures for alcohol intake in 32 countries for which reliable figures are available.

TABLE 4.1
Per capita figures for alcohol intake in countries for which figures are available

Country	Litres	Country	Litres
Luxembourg	21.0	Netherlands	11.3
France	19.2	United States	11.2
Portugal	18.1	Ireland	10.4
Spain	17.6	Romania	10.3
East Germany	16.0	Yugoslavia	10.2
West Germany	15.7	Bulgaria	9.9
Hungary	15.6	United Kingdom	9.3
Switzerland	14.1	Poland	8.7
Czechoslovakia	14.1	Finland	8.3
Austria	14.0	USSR	8.2
Australia	13.9	Japan	7.8
Italy	13.7	Sweden	6.8
Belgium	13.2	Norway	5.3
Denmark	12.8	Iceland	5.2
New Zealand	12.5	Mexico	5.0
Canada	11.4	Israel	3.1

Source: International Survey, Alcoholic Beverage Taxation and Control Policies, Fifth Edition, Brewers Association of Canada, 1981

The relative standings of these nations do not change radically from one year to the next, although there has been a general and noticeable rise in intake and alcohol problems in recent years in the industrialised world.[3] The figures relate to per capita intake and not problem drinking (for which reliable figures are not readily available), though the two are not unrelated. Exceptions to the figures in Table 4.1 are the relative rates of alcohol problems in Ireland and Italy. Ireland has a lower per capita intake than Italy but, by common consent, higher rates of alcoholism. The evidence is that differences amongst ethnic groups are stable over time.

An early example is the rejection rates for alcohol problems in military recruits in the Boston area during the Second World War.[4] The rejection rate of Irish-Americans was twice that of

Italian-Americans, and 15 times greater than that of Americans from a Jewish background. Forty years later Muhlin[5] reported on the differences between alcohol problems for Irish and Italian residents in psychiatric facilities in New York State. He found that over 50 per cent of the Irish men, but only 4 per cent of the Italian men, were hospitalised with alcohol-related diagnoses. Muhlin entitled his paper 'Ethnic differences in alcohol misuse: a striking reaffirmation', and clearly there are significant and persistent differences in alcohol abuse between ethnic groups. From where do these differences arise? In descriptive terms, the most important factor is whether the individual in question has a family history of problem drinking.

The interpretation of these obvious differences is no simple matter. Early writers saw the differences as rooted in nature rather than nurture. At the turn of the century Crothers wrote that 'the heredity of inebriety is established beyond all possible doubt'.[6] Subsequent research data on this point have not been at all what Crothers would have hoped. To quote again from the 1983 review of Saunders and Williams: 'Studies of adopted children and of monozygotic [identical] compared with dizygotic [fraternal] twins show a modest but definite genetic influence on drinking habits . . . [and] no biological markers have been associated convincingly with a predisposition to alcoholism'. Where the biological offspring of mothers with alcohol problems raised by non-alcoholic adoptive parents show a raised incidence compared with controls, environmental factors may still play a role in the form of influences on the foetus in the intrauterine environment. Apart from the adverse effects of alcohol abuse during pregnancy, there are studies which reveal that mammals exposed to alcohol *in utero* and/or during breast feeding have increased preferences for alcohol in later life, as well as learning difficulties and hyperactivity.[7]

A hypothesis borrowed from the field of schizophrenia may help to suggest the ways in which genetic and environmental factors impact upon one another to influence the course of development. First proposed by Paul Meehl, it addressed two well-established findings about schizophrenia. The first is that twin studies comparing monozygotic and dizygotic twins always show a higher concordance rate for the former over the latter. In line with these findings, adoption studies reveal that children of schizophrenic mothers and/or fathers raised by non-schizophrenic adoptive parents are more like their biological than their adoptive parents. In general, the sheer amount of the data from a variety of sources[8] amounts to incontrovertible evidence for the heritability of schizophrenia. However, set against these findings are the failures ever to find perfect concordance between pairs of monozygotic twins and, second, substantial numbers of the offspring of schizophrenic parents who are raised by adoptive parents and who escape clinical schizophrenia, thereby establishing a case for habit and culture in schizophrenia.

Meehl constructed a stress-diathesis model to accommodate the two sets of findings. A diathesis, the inherited vulnerability, is not by itself sufficient to produce schizophrenia. A vulnerable person raised in a benign environment and/or who is equipped with the requisite coping skills to manage the demands placed upon him would not decompensate to a psychotic condition. For a person without the diathesis no amount of stress and adversity would eventuate in a diagnosis of schizophrenia (but might lead to a different disorder, with its own specific diathesis). When applied to alcoholism the stress-diathesis model allows for the heritability of a predisposition to excessive drinking (or to the chance of greater organ damage in the wake of excessive drinking) but does not concede to a fully genetic account of alcoholism. Information as to the exact nature of the diathesis is scanty, but there is practical value in the stress-diathesis account of chronic alcohol problems. Sufficient evidence now exists on the risks of familial alcoholism to justify counselling total abstinence to those with a strong history of highly heritable forms of dependence or susceptibility to physical damage from heavy drinking.

More is known about the environmental factors that may potentiate the diathesis, or which can directly promote drinking in their own right. Of these, 'modelling' influences and expectations stimulated a great amount of research which is of considerable importance to clinical practice.

In psychology, modelling is the study of interpersonal influences on behaviour, cognitions and emotions. Earlier, in the discussion of drinking, alcohol problems and ethnic/religious groups, it was noted that Jews in Israel and Americans of Jewish origin drank much less than Irish Americans. That there are modelling effects at work here is suggested by studies which show that as the religious affiliations of Jews alter from orthodox, to conservative, to secular, signs of alcohol problems increase markedly.[9] In Orthodox Jewish custom the use of alcohol is permitted but strictly circumscribed by ceremonial practice. As those of Jewish background integrate with non-Jewish society so they begin to display drinking practices and problems which resemble those of their new, heavier drinking companions.

Controlled laboratory demonstrations of modelling show the direct influence of the drinking behaviour of companions on a person's alcohol intake in 'normal' and 'heavy' drinkers. Subjects in a study by Caudill et al.[10] were recruited from a population of university student volunteers. The experimenters wished to assess the effect of heavy or light drinking models on the drinking behaviour of their subjects. One serious obstacle faced them. Had their real intentions been announced the subjects might have displayed a self-serving moderation (and in so doing avoided the twin stigmas of 'alcoholic' and 'lacking in willpower'). To guard against such threats to the validity of the experiment the subjects were deceived as to its true purpose, being told that they were to take part in a 'taste test'. Wine was given them to drink and to rate on a number of scales as to whether it was bitter, salty and so on, and they were asked to drink as much or as little as they needed to make their ratings. The real target of interest was the amount of wine they consumed, measured after they had left the room. Each of the subjects took the 'taste test' with one 'fellow student' who was, unbeknownst to them, actually a research confederate. Half the subjects were exposed to a model who drank heavily while making his 'ratings', while the other half were exposed to a light drinking model. Those who had the heavy drinking model in the room with them consumed significantly more wine while making their own 'ratings' than did those who took the test along with a light drinking 'fellow student'.

A straightforward interpretation of these data is that the amount of alcohol we consume is influenced by the drinking behaviour of those with whom we associate. If this is the case, then the belief that we consciously choose how much we drink requires reexamination.

Let us now consider work done in this vein but carried out in the natural environment. Changes in the drinking practices of

Jewish people which coincide with the patterns of drinking in their families and friends supply no more than correlational data. One complementary finding is missing from the findings discussed thus far: experiments in naturalistic settings. Collins et al. supplied this information in a 1985 report.[11] Men whose drinking behaviour was observed (covertly) in taverns showed a significant tendency to match the consumption of models in both heavy and light drinking conditions. An unexpected finding was that 'matching' was observed only when the models behaved in a warm and friendly way. When the model's behaviour (which was regulated according to instructions given by the experimenter beforehand) was 'cold and unsociable' the subjects drank at a high rate, regardless of the model's rate of consumption. The experimenters speculate that 'subjects in the "light-model consumption unsociable" condition might have consumed more beer in an effort to cope with the threat of being unable to establish rapport with an unresponsive partner'. The idea of heightened alcohol consumption occurring as a (maladaptive) reaction to distressing emotional states is in line with a host of findings linking relapse to loss of self-esteem in negative emotional situations.[12]

Looking back on these results it would be premature to assume that modelling effects are simply a form of imitation. Emotional pressure exerts a strong influence on alcohol intake, as do the social characteristics of the model. Returning to the 'taste test' experiment, it is entirely possible that the heavy drinking models caused the subjects to feel under pressure to 'keep up' with their 'fellow students' so as to show that they, too, could 'hold their liquor'. Admittedly this is going beyond the facts as reported by Caudill et al., but anecdotal evidence strongly suggests that peer pressure can be a powerful determinant in substance abuse problems. The clinical implications for assessment and therapy are: obtain a clear estimate of the drinking practices and attitudes of the patient's drinking companions and family, and if they model and/or urge heavy drinking the patient must (a) learn first to be aware of this and then (b) learn the most socially appropriate means of carrying through with firm counter-pressure assertive skills. These might be less important for heavily dependent drinkers once drinking has already begun. For such individuals, for whom abstinence is essential, assertive skills are best directed at refusing pressures to begin a bout of drinking in the first place.

Controlled drinkers would require assistance in being able to resist the pressures to continue drinking once they have reached a sensible limit.

If the literature on modelling and alcohol consumption makes intuitive sense, popular expectations about the effects of alcohol on feeling states produced by excessive drinking are at dramatic odds with the evidence on alcohol and its effects. Alcohol is assumed to function as a potent but habit-forming and dangerous liquid tranquilliser: 'It has long been recognised that tension, stress, anxiety and related physical and psychological states are frequently unpleasant or painful for the organism and much of our behaviour is motivated by the need to eliminate or reduce those sensations or feelings . . . Any activity which [for example, gulping alcohol] . . . has the desired effect—reduction of or elimination of unpleasant stimuli—is rewarding or reinforcing, and therefore the probability of that activity or event is increased, so that the next time the individual experiences the unpleasant stimuli he or she is increasingly more likely to employ the alcohol-drinking response'. It is not difficult to imagine, then, that the 'alcohol-drinking response' soon occurs in anticipation of unpleasant experiences. Gradually, it is assumed, one finds that the alcohol-drinking response has become necessary for daily functioning[13]—to keep anxiety and depression at bay.[14]

Teenagers, the general public and patients all have these expectations about 'what drinking alcohol does to, and for, you'. Though at first glance plausible, are they valid assumptions? Patients certainly believe so.[15,16] In the available evidence positive expectations were shown to be held without reservation. In striking contrast, the effects of alcohol consumption were dramatically at odds with these expectations. In reviewing the published reports Mello,[17] speaking of her results and those from similar research, wrote: 'The voluminous literature on alcoholism has often tended to present "the alcoholic" as an impulsive hedonist who drinks to dissolve his anxieties and achieve a diffuse sense of omnipotence. Direct observations of intoxicated alcoholics have revealed a pathetic failure to attain such goals.' Note that the focus in these studies is how problem drinkers seem to others and report themselves to be *as they move through the drinking bout.*

Paredes reports identical outcomes: 'Interestingly, patients who drank experienced increasing subjective discomfort' (i.e. when asked to give self-evaluations they made it clear that they were experiencing dysphoria, not its opposite). Paredes adds 'This type of evidence has challenged the adequacy of a tension-reducing model of alcoholism'.[18] He has fallen into a common but unfortunate confusion here. 'Tension' is not a synonym for mood, anxiety or depression. In the experiments he mentions, mood was, but tension was not, measured. Indeed it is tension—in the sense of muscle tension—that is affected positively by alcohol. Steffen et al.[19] did find tension reduction in a group of male alcoholics, but they also found an increase in mood disturbance at the same time. Hence there is support for a *tension* reduction but not for an anxiety-depression-dysphoria reduction hypothesis.

In one of the most dramatic counter-examples to the stress alleviation hypothesis, Tamerin et al.[20] obtained the expectations from alcoholics of what they thought they would experience when drinking. The subjects expected and predicted positive mood changes. They were then allowed to have an experimental 'free drinking' session, which lasted from 14 to 60 days. During the drinking sessions the subjects demonstrated more aggression than they had predicted prior to each session and yet experienced significant declines in mood while drinking. Despite this 'mismatch', during post-experimental questioning on the following day the drinkers reaffirmed their expectations that alcohol would affect them positively on the next occasion when they drank.

One possible answer to this extraordinary persistence of positive expectations is that the initial but short-lived euphoria of the first few drinks is all that is recalled 'the morning after'. It is conceivable that alcoholic 'blackouts' might obscure from subsequent recall the events and feelings of the middle and latter parts of the drinking bout. The experimenters report that blackouts were common. This would allow the highly unpleasant mood and behaviour changes to be hidden behind an amnesiac barrier, leaving the positive expectancies intact.

The mismatch between the persistent beliefs about alcohol and the emotional reactions observed during extended drinking (dysphoria) is a matter of clinical concern. Since expectancies can have an important influence on drinking practices, the patient's attitudes and awareness must be probed and, where necessary, modified. Clinicians who assume, without question, that alcohol is an anxiolytic can no longer justify this belief. The link between anxiety (or depression) and alcohol is one in which alcohol can be seen as a substance which causes, induces or intensifies emotional problems: 'while excessive alcohol use causing depression runs counter to the layman's view that alcohol alleviates depression, laboratory studies . . . as well as cross sectional clinical and longitudinal studies of alcoholics all support the proposition that high doses of alcohol can induce depressive affect, at least in individuals who have alcohol problems of dependence'.[21]

Much the same conclusion applies to the effect of alcohol on preexisting anxiety disorders. In a 1986 paper Thyer and his associates examined 156 consecutive admissions meeting *DSM III* criteria for agoraphobia, panic reactions, social phobia or generalised anxiety disorder. Approximately 20 per cent scored in the alcoholic range on the Michigan Alcoholism Screening Test. When the effects of alcohol on such anxiety disorders were estimated 'periods of heavy drinking and dependence upon alcohol were associated with an *exacerbation* of agoraphobia and social phobias'[22] (emphasis added).

There is another paradox in addition to the one just discussed. This is the belief that stress—in whatever form—produces an inclination to seek out alcohol to obtain relief from stress. It is assumed that as life's stresses mount and finally overtax the drinker's defences he 'turns to drink'. Alcohol is said to work only too well, causing the drinker to rely on it increasingly, until finally it produces an 'addiction'. We know now that the second part of this robust piece of folk wisdom is fundamentally wrong. But the first part, which states that psychological stress can lead to excessive drinking, is supported. In one study, eight alcoholics and eight social drinkers were allowed to work a lever to obtain alcohol. Prior to a period of stress both the alcoholics and the social drinkers responded at comparable rates. The stress period required the subjects in both groups to role-play assertive responses in five difficult social situations. The subjects found the role playing, with critical social feedback, stressful. This was seen in the pulse rate data, which showed a significant increase in both groups. But while 100 per cent of the alcoholics increased their lever pressing so as to obtain more alcohol, only a quarter of the control group showed an increase.[23]

The data from the study of clinical relapse tell a similar story.

Approximately 60 per cent of a group of alcoholics who had taken part in an aversion therapy treatment relapsed following frustrating, anger-eliciting or socially stressful challenges. In a recently published book on relapse prevention, Marlatt and Gordon[24] mention studies of their own, and of others, which reveal that stressful encounters with significant others are followed by a return to problem drinking. By contrast, non social stressors (threats of electric shock) are of little significance and lead to few, if any, changes in drinking.

To summarise, social stressors can lead to drinking, but the drinking, contrary to theories of reinforcement or plain common sense, does not feed back to alleviate the stress it produces in the first place. Paradoxically, in problem drinkers heavy drinking can and does exacerbate the problems that lead to drinking. The cycle is not apparent to the drinker. Faulty expectations and the varieties of modelling influences are two important processes to be monitored and modified in treating problem drinking.

CHAPTER 5

Why Treatments Fail: 'Lack of Motivation' and 'Denial'

'Probably in no other illness is so much verbal concern manifested in the patient's motivation to recover as in alcoholism.'[1] In a survey of why treatments fail, 75 per cent of the treatment personnel surveyed replied that lack of motivation to improve was an important factor; for 50 per cent the presence of motivation was the prerequisite for recovery.[2] Problem drinkers are perceived as especially unmotivated, compared with all other patients. The explanation for this is supposed to be that, unlike other patients, alcoholics derive more pleasure than distress from engaging in their habit: 'no alcoholic will consider abstaining until alcohol brings more suffering than pleasure'.[3] The corollary is that unless extraordinary steps are taken there will be no change and treatments will fail.

The explanation most commonly advanced to account for the assumed failure of motivation to change, and thus of the poor prognosis of problem drinkers, is that they have developed a web of defence mechanisms by which they fool themselves and attempt to fool others. Denial is a malignant process common to all alcoholics. Says Fox, a spokesperson for the defenders of orthodoxy: 'patients refuse to face their alcoholism for many years, using the defense mechanisms of denial, rationalization, regression and projection'.[4] Were it not for these pathological defence systems, and the alcoholic's character disorders, treatments would succeed. At least that was the belief found most often by Moore[5] in his nation-wide US survey. Seventy-two per cent of clinicians working with alcoholics blamed failures on the patients, while 11 per cent admitted that the way the patients were treated might have something to do with negative outcomes. Alcoholics Anonymous, too, explain lack of motivation by indicting the drinker: 'Rarely have we seen a person fail who has thoroughly followed our path. Those who do not recover are people who cannot or will not completely give themselves to this simple program, usually men and women who are *constitutionally incapable* of being honest with themselves'[6] (emphasis added).

The wide acceptance gained by these explanations may help to explain why, in a survey of psychiatrists, 89 per cent described problem drinkers as 'more difficult', 'much more difficult' and even 'impossible' to treat, when compared with other psychiatric cases.[7] It also suggests why it is believed by most health professionals that drastic steps must be taken if there is to be any hope of recovery. These steps will inevitably cause suffering and even then may not work until the drinker 'hits rock bottom'. Patients must be pressured and 'undergo the processes of surrender and reduction of ego'.[8] The gamut of popular techniques and counter-reactions to denial runs from fear-inducing lectures to harsh confrontation methods.

Miller's excellent 1985 review of motivation for treatment[9] cites an example reported in 1983 by Greenburger[10] which gives a feel of the confrontation 'techniques' deliberately engineered to 'break' the drinker's denial. The situation described was a confrontation intervention in a programme for employees with drinking problems: 'They called a surprise meeting (with the alcoholic), surrounded him with colleagues critical of his work and threatened to fire him if he didn't seek help quickly. When the executive tried to deny that he had a drinking problem the medical director . . . came down hard. "Shut up and listen," he said. "Alcoholics are liars, so we don't want to hear what you have to say".'[11] Why such abrupt and aggressive behaviour? The reasons given are stated in terms of the evasions said to be present in all problem drinkers: 'The layers of denial in alcoholism [which] run deep . . . present an almost impenetrable wall'[12] to the entreaties of the therapist.

Viewing the system from outside, it is tempting to wonder if charges of denial and interventions of therapeutic hostility (for surely they must appear more hostile than helpful to the patient) are not defences employed by the clinician. They do, after all, provide ready-made excuses for the three difficulties which bedevil the exasperated clinician: dropouts, failures and post-abstinence relapses ('falling off the wagon'). But rather than set forth a new set of accusations, it would be of more use to search for explanations for these problems and the techniques to manage them.

In the search for the basis of 'motivation', two contrasting approaches have been employed. Traditionalists assert the existence of personality differences between drinkers who stay in and those who drop out of treatment programmes.[13] There is indeed some evidence for 'personality defects' in the alcoholics who drop out which reveal 'denial' and 'hostility'. When looked at from another angle, however, a different picture emerges. If motivational interpretations are ways of estimating the probability of behaviour change occuring within an inter-personal context, the questions to ask are: 'hostility to whom?' and 'denial of what?' If the answers are: 'hostility to those I do not trust who attack me,' and 'denial that I am a "hopeless drunk" ', then the problem lies in the relationship between the therapist and the patient, and not in the patient alone.

Compliance and maintaining contact

We mentioned in Chapter 1 that most problem drinkers are not detected until the consequences of alcohol abuse have taken a serious toll. The regular use of screening and assessment measures (see Chapter 6) can go a long way towards dealing with failures of detection. However, even when problem drinkers are detected and referred to a treatment facility, the bulk of them never attend, or if they do, come for a session or two only. Inconsistent attendance is taken as further proof of denial. 'It's now up to them' seems to be the general attitude towards the drinker's motivation, once his problem has been detected and a referral has been given. However, when direct but non-intrusive methods are used to enhance contact and attendance, dramatic improvements in 'motivation' have been found. A 1962 study found that only 5 per cent of alcoholics seen in a large urban hospital were successfully referred to an alcoholic clinic. This figure was raised to 65 per cent, an exceptional increase, simply by having the patient seen by a psychiatrist or the hospital social worker. In another, later study, when the first-contact counsellor took the responsibility for placing the referral call to the alcohol clinic the completion rate was 82 per cent; if it was left to the client to phone the figure was significantly lower (37 per cent).

Another means of motivating the patient to attend the initial session is to shorten the delay between telephone contact and the first session at the clinic. The longer the prospective patient is asked to wait the lower the chance that he will attend when an appointment is finally arranged.[14] Once the patient attends it is vital that steps be taken to increase his motivation to return. A research study which took up this question yielded very positive results from a small amount of effort.[15] Patients who received a letter from the clinic offering a new appointment after they had missed a second or subsequent appointment were less likely to discontinue therapy (28 per cent) than a control group (51 per cent) not sent reminder letters. As the authors of this study interpreted their results, patients who expected pessimistic rejection and who instead received a sign of genuine concern became more motivated to continue: 'The more the therapist is seen as wanting to help the patient, the more the patient will be motivated to continue the relationship'.[16]

Jacobs believes that a letter is, in most instances, preferable to a telephone call. He describes the ideal letter as being neutral and nonjudgmental. A telephone call, no matter how well intentioned, is likely to put the client on the defensive, making him feel that an explanation is necessary, even when none has been asked for.[17] Jacobs may be right, or it may be that the content of the communication and not the form of the contact is the crucial variable. Research on the question favours the latter position. When they were compared, both letters and phone contacts were shown to be successful, whereas an impersonal letter had no effect on continuity of attendance. Koumans et al. compared 50 patients who did and 50 who did not receive a follow-up telephone call after their first visit to a treatment clinic.[18] The return rate for the contact group was 44 per cent, compared with 8 per cent for the non-contact group.

The above findings fit poorly with the prevailing attitudes denigrating drinkers for lacking motivation and the habit of mind which assigns all responsibility for change to the patient. Where an effort is made to communicate care to the drinker/patient quite exceptional increases can be expected in patient 'motivation', at least as regards initial attendance.

These findings may still fail to impress some people: whether or not a problem drinker attends clinical sessions may seem to them to be a small matter. It is possible to retain traditional trait-attributions about denial while admitting that actual attendance can be enhanced by changes in clinical practice. It might be argued that the clinical outcome is all-important, a good outcome depending on enhancing motivation to stop drinking, which in turn rests on bringing the drinker face-to-face with his denial.

The negative attitude towards alcoholics held by non-specialist clinicians across a variety of professions has already been noted. Interestingly, if experienced clinicians, problem drinkers and new trainees are surveyed it is in the attitudes of the more experienced professionals that the most pessimism is found towards the alcoholic and his prognosis. The usual explanation offered for this pattern is that the positive attitudes of the fledgling therapists is simple 'over optimism'. It is commonly held that with extended contacts novice clinicians will shift towards 'realism'. In practice this seems to mean a readiness to evaluate the drinker's 'real' motivations negatively and a greater resort to confrontational methods to attack the basic problems—denial, lack of motivation and the impulsive hedonism of all alcoholics. There is nothing faulty in the logic of this argument: its drawback lies in the negativity of outlook it fosters. Can therapists afford to ignore the impact of their attitudes on the patient? More exactly, do clinical outcomes depend on therapist expectancies?

When therapist expectancies about patients are deliberately, and covertly, manipulated, clinical outcomes are in line with induced expectations.[19] In a study by Leake and his co-workers counsellors were informed that, on the basis of certain tests, one group of problem drinkers would turn out to be punctual, highly motivated to accept treatment and would make more of an effort on their own behalf. A different group was described as ordinary alcoholics with no special attributes. This was a deception, as no tests had been given, the drinkers having been randomly assigned to the 'good prognosis' or 'ordinary' condition. The descriptions of patient motivation worked in the expected direction. The 'good prognosis' patients were absent from therapy significantly less often and fewer terminated treatment programmes. Most importantly, assessment showed that the 'special' patients had more sober days at one-year follow-up.

Exactly why those randomly allocated to the bogus 'good' group not only stayed longer in therapy but actually improved more on drinking measures as well is a matter for speculation. A plausible guess is that a virtuous rather than a vicious cycle was set up by the subtle manipulation of therapist expectancies. It would have begun with the therapists translating their positive expectancies into supportive and empathic behaviour. The circular and desirable pattern would have been completed by an increase in the patients' self-esteem and cooperation with the clinical personnel. Lowered self-esteem and counter hostility is a reaction to fear tactics and a potent cause of self-defeating, defensive, dependent and avoidance behaviour.[20] Conversely, high self-esteem, which is fostered by respect and courtesy (amongst other things) is associated with positive change and a reduction in alcohol problems.

Left as it is, it would appear that we are fixing the blame for failures or the reasons for successes entirely upon 'non-specific' factors like the patient's feelings of support and the clinician's belief in the possibility of change for the better. Indeed, there are writers who go further to assert, in our view mistakenly, that one therapy is as good as any other, as long as it is founded upon a good working relationship and 'mutual empathy' in the therapist-patient interaction.[21] Those who are attracted to the idea that good relationships and positive expectancies are sufficient, consider specific techniques essentially as 'placebos'. We disagree. Evidence indicating the effectiveness of empathy and persistence in promoting attendance is of value in framing remedies for dropout problems and non-compliance. However, the drinking disorders themselves require knowledge of a host of factors from dependence to coexisting psychiatric problems. 'Being nice' is not enough.

Techniques for treating alcoholism have been investigated extensively; the behaviour of the therapist in coping with 'difficult' or misguided patients has been neglected by researchers and undervalued by practitioners. This state of affairs is due in large part ot the absence of systematic concern with the treatment of motivational deficits, the identification of common misunderstandings and the approach to 'denials' in the university training of clinicians. Dean's complaint made in 1958 still holds today: 'Graduate schools do not offer courses on the treatment of the reluctant client ... [hence] psychotherapy proceeds from the assumption of a motivated client', which may in the clinical reality be far from the truth. First on the agenda is the answer to this question: 'What are the techniques most likely to produce motivation in what kinds of reluctant client?'

If we understand 'reluctance' to mean that the newly arrived patient is caught between pressures to continue his drinking habits and the fear of negative evaluation and his desire to rid himself of his afflictions, then our goal must be to find the approach and techniques which tip the balance away from fear and in favour of change. This process begins with the very first interview and goes on to include information giving, skills acquisition (from problem solving to tension management), attitude (cognitive) change, incentive modification and relapse therapy.

Every stage in the process depends on the patient's self-reports about drinking and problems connected with it. The validity of the self-reports rest on the patient's willingness, and ability, to give undistorted answers. So great are the doubts expressed in clinical writings about accurate self-reports that in some quarters behavioural observations and medical tests are preferred in principle to the patient's verbal responses. Though medical data and, where possible, controlled behavioural observations can provide valuable information, the idea that a collection of objective behavioural and medical facts can eliminate the need for reliance upon the patient's reports fails to recognise the central significance of the patient's perspective on the outcome of therapy. Medical data on, say, liver functioning, cannot establish trust between patient and therapist; careful observations of drinking behaviour are beside the point if the patient persists in defensive denials. Nor can a medical examination substitute for information relating to the details of drinking episodes and their emotional consequences. Inevitably, the clinician will have to rely upon the patient's own statements about his drinking, and the patient's thoughts and feelings about others, himself and alcohol. The clinician can turn to people close to the patient for corroboration but these data are not error-free either. Reports of drinking behaviour given by relatives may be more distorted or inaccurate than estimates given by drinkers themselves. The reports of relatives and friends must also be evaluated; they are not direct avenues to 'the truth'.

Dealing with denials

We are thus back where we began, with clinician and patient talking to each other in the interview. The word interview as used here refers to the complex of interactions which are initiated in the very first meeting and which conclude with the termination of the relationship between therapist and patient. If the information obtained in 'the interview' is discarded or if the patient's self-reports are discounted, access is lost to vital material that is otherwise unobtainable. This is self-evident, but from a reading of the clinical literature over the last 20 years it is also evident that there are deep reservations about the truth of the patient's statements (by those of the traditional orientations; behavioural clinicians have barely paid any attention to the issue).

It is a truism in these writings that alcoholics are unmotivated and unreliable patients. Denial, inconsistent attendance, poor cooperation with clinical rules and requests and premature termination are mentioned as the most serious manifestations of a motivational deficit which resides within the personality of 'the alcoholic'. Of these, denial has been the subject of most discussion and is considered to be the significant barrier to rehabilitation. The treatment corollary is that before all else, steps must be taken to weaken denial. What these should be is still a matter for speculation. For a problem accorded the status of first priority, denial has yet to be studied scientificially. After years of discussion there is not even consensus on the precise definition of denial. We find the one used by Forrest captures the essential feature of denial: the refusal to acknowledge the degree of control that alcohol has assumed in the drinker's life. The reasons for the persistence of denial can vary from one patient to the next, and there is no reason to believe that there will ever be one definitive strategy which will apply in all cases. What can be stated with a measure of confidence is that the resort to forceful confrontations with the drinker, a practice endemic in traditional programmes, is positively correlated with treatment failure. Hostile confrontations are to be avoided at all times, whether the hostility is expressed in words or tone. In a convincing demonstration of this point researchers took the verbal content of nine doctors and compared the transcripts with treatment outcome. Ratings of the verbal content were unrelated to outcome, but when the taped interviews were passed through a filter which rendered the verbal content unintelligible it allowed the 'blind' clinical judges to hear the emotional content of the exchanges. Ratings of hostility in the voices of doctors were a significant predictor of treatment success or failure ($r=.65$).

What then can be done about denial? A useful first step which has been proposed by Jacobs is to distinguish 'genuine' from 'public' deniers. Genuine deniers do not admit the existence of a problem to others or to themselves; public deniers privately acknowledge problems with alcohol. From the treatment of denial in the clinical literature the former are assumed to make up the majority of deniers, but until any evidence is available the utility of the category must be regarded as speculative. Public deniers are likely to respond to supportive and non-judgmental discussions. The clinician should reply to denial with suggestions like: 'it might be helpful if we discussed your drinking,' or 'it might be time to cut down on your drinking'. If the patient disagrees, the therapist can focus the discussion on the times and places when drinking goes beyond reasonable limits: 'are there particular situations when you are likely to drink more than is sensible?'; 'Why do you think your wife is so concerned about your drinking?'

If 'denial' continues the therapist should consider the possibility that the patient has a different set of criteria for his own assessment of problem drinking from those adopted by the therapist. In such cases the word 'disagreement' is preferable to 'denial'. The most profitable course would then be to probe for the existence of misunderstandings about the patient's conclusions or misinformation about what constitutes an alcohol problem. Patients may erroneously believe that the only risk is drinking to the point of intoxication, or that only spirits (whisky, vodka and so on) are dangerous, or that all problem drinkers live on Skid Row.

The therapist must also guard against treatments of denial or disagreement which require the patient to accept the label 'alcoholic', with its connotations of personal helplessness. Patients who acquiesce to the 'sick role' (and the associated belief that they are unable to overcome their problems with planning and volitional control) are rated by staff as more enjoyable to work with but are less likely to take an active part in behaviour-change programmes.

The therapist who takes reasonable steps to promote higher levels of motivation, lower levels of denial, and to resolve disagreements, will encounter some patients who insist, in the face of massive evidence to the contrary, that drinking is no problem in their lives. Medical evidence or statements of concern (not accusations) by those close to the patient may help to soften resistance. However, with some there will come a time when matters cannot be allowed to continue to drift aimlessly. Equally serious mismatches, if uncorrected, inevitably lead to the termination of therapy.

Mismatches can be held to a minimum if commonsense guidelines and ordinary courtesies are observed. The three areas set out below are ones that we rehearse to ourselves before seeing a patient.

Courtesy in the initial interaction The patient seeking help for drinking problems will have formed expectancies in two areas—about his problems and about the response he is likely to encounter in the clinician. Both will be coloured by the attitudes of society towards alcoholism and he will be aware that they are overwhelmingly negative. Though he may strenuously resist the diagnosis of 'alcoholism' his very presence is an admission that he cannot control his drinking and/or that others have impressed that unpalatable fact upon him. It is safe to begin with the assumption that he will be highly ambivalent about seeking help, possibly demoralised and almost certainly defensive. Griffith Edwards[22] asks the clinician 'to be keenly aware of this and to be careful that he is not taking his own good-will as self-evident. The clinician should make his positive attitude clear and overt. From the first special care must be put into showing ordinary courtesies; to walk up the corridor with the patient rather than five paces in front . . . to show him towards a comfortable chair are . . . small but telling gestures.' Other courtesies are addressing the patient as Mr, Mrs or Ms and not by first name unless invited to do so, and refraining from using the words 'girl' or 'lass' when talking to or of women.

Confidentiality After relaxed but thoughtful demonstrations of courtesy the patient must be directly and immediately assured of confidentiality. This, too, might seem self-evident, but the patient may harbour suspicions of the therapist giving out personal details of his drinking and emotional problems. Assurances should be given that no information will be divulged to anyone for any reason without the patient's consent. His worries are not to be shunted aside as the preoccupations of a neurotic: people do stereotype alcoholics negatively and there will be few patients unaware of this. Moreover, we know of many instances of health-care professionals discussing referral possibilities and the details of a patient's disorder without mentioning to that patient whom they had contacted or what had been said. While in defence they are likely to reply that they had the patient's interest at heart, this is beside the point.

To calm the patient's apprehensions, as soon as the initial pleasantries are concluded we recommend that time be taken to give the strongest reassurances, in this sort of form:

> 'Before we begin on what you'd like to talk about I should like to say that any matters that we may discuss will be treated in the strictest confidence. Nothing that we say or do here will be made known to anyone unless we both agree that it will be of help to you to do so. I emphasise this because I believe that we can do the best possible work together if we are in agreement on this and all other important matters. Whatever direction we decide therapy should take, rest assured that I am opposed to the use of "surprise tactics" or taking any steps before we discuss the best ways of managing problems. I am stressing these points not because I believe that your concerns are unusual or that I see them as a stigma to be concealed. Getting into difficulties with alcohol is far from a rare thing. My promise of confidentiality is simply another way of saying that if we are going to get anywhere together we must work in collaboration.'

A summary of this chapter can be given in a few sentences. 'Difficult' patients, treatment casualties, dropouts and relapses have plagued clinicians working with alcoholics. Over the years explanations have tagged these as a function of motivational deficits and 'denials', symptoms of an intrinsic pathology in all alcoholics.

A radical alternative to orthodox methods challenges the traditional perspective in two ways. First, rather than categorising motivation as a 'thing' which exists in full measure or is absent altogether, the likelihood of cooperation (motivation) can be described as falling along a continuum from very low to very high. Second, and following on from this, modifications to therapeutic practice and attitudes can now be recognised as powerful determinants of motivation, which *can* be raised if the right conditions are created. Motivation is as much 'in' the environment and 'in' the relationship which the therapist and patient establish, as it is 'in' the patient. Seeing it exclusively as a property of the patient fosters pessimism in some clinicians and encourages others to search for even more powerful forms of confrontation. In either of these directions lie more denials, dropouts and failures. These may happen anyway (for example, with patients who come to treatment clinics under legal coercion) but the risks are far greater if pessimism and hostility are present.

CHAPTER 6

Assessment

For years assessment has been a routine of clinical practice and a negligible part of therapy. The usual ordering of events was (and still is) for the patient to be tested soon after entry into the clinical facility, and once put through the usual battery of tests to be sent elsewhere in the clinic to be treated according to the usual practice favoured in that clinic. Apart from supplying the therapist with a few summary estimates of intelligence and personality functioning, the assessment results were generally filed and forgotten. Information concerning changes in day-to-day functioning and movements towards, or away, from adaptive changes may or may not have been noted, but were not systematically incorporated into the treatment programme. Narrow, ultra-behavioural, clinicians focussed on the externals ('How many drinks did you have yesterday?'; 'Where and when did you have them?'), while analytic therapists directed their enquiries to the symptomatic manifestations of the 'inner' dynamics of deep personality disorders. For those who worked within a psychoanalytical framework, information as to the number of drinks consumed yesterday, if of interest at all, was taken to be but one more surface symptom of the real disorder lying deep within the unconscious.

Neither of these two approaches is satisfactory, but the behavioural 'drink counters' did at least concern themselves with important objective data, whereas the employment of projective tests to measure poorly defined personality dynamics ('ego strength'; 'dependancy needs'; 'changes in superego functioning') favoured the use of poorly defined and global clinical inferences about hypothetical psychodynamic impulses and defences. Though these continue to feature in clinical practice, broad generalisations of this kind have been shown to be deficient in reliability, validity and utility and thus are of no value in serious assessment programmes. Current evaluations are beginning to reflect this judgement: in a recent handbook of assessment

Auerbach[1] delivered a harsh judgement on the practice of centering assessment on global qualities which are interpreted as disguised symptoms of unconscious conflicts: 'If ever . . . [such assumptions and conclusions] were able to command the agreement of the majority of therapists that day . . . [should be] past.'

Increasingly the contemporary trend is for the use of continuous methods of assessment which interlink with change techniques to form the basis of the therapeutic programme. Evidence strongly favours the case that if the patient is to make real improvements, his active collaboration must be elicited. Hence the patient who comes for help with problems cannot be treated as someone who can be expected to, first, give answers to questions and then to follow instructions as given. It is now increasingly accepted that assessment is not a 'one time thing' but an ongoing process involving the sympathetic cooperation of both members of the therapeutic team: patient and clinician. Its basic purposes are to estimate risk factors for problem drinking, to establish goals and priorities, and to monitor the effects of behaviour-change programmes. The risk areas are: (a) risk for alcohol abuse and dependence, (b) risk for the clinical consequences of excessive drinking, and (c) risk for psychiatric and social problems linked to drinking.

Ideally, measures developed to assess the patient's functioning 'must be concise, communicable and quantifiable . . . based on factual data that can be observed reliably by more than one individual'.[2] Inevitably the practical realities of assessment differ somewhat as clinicians must, in the main, rely on the patient's self-reports which are subject to defensive distortion, the vagaries of recall and the misunderstandings and biases which form the patients' theory about what is wrong and what is to be done about it.

As has already been stated, there are no ready-made solutions for the communication problems which can arise between patient and therapist. In the main these can be managed if the therapist reminds himself to avoid the twin pitfalls of pessimism and hostility. When faced with deceptions, backsliding and 'failures' therapists can become ensnared in their own frustrations and may lose sight of the patient's needs and fears. If so the worst motivations can be imputed to the patient ('He doesn't want to change!'). Inadequacies are misconstrued as contrariness, and lies told about drinking under fear of rejection are taken as evidence of a capricious game-playing mentality on the part of the patient. The counter-reactions of pessimism and hostility by the therapist, disguised as 'hard-headed realism' and 'direct confrontation' are understandable but totally counterproductive. While we are unaware of any evidence bearing on the prevalence of these reactions, it is our impression that therapists who work with alcohol and other drug patients are especially prone to them. These errors were discussed in Chapter 5.

Another serious mistake is to divorce assessment from therapy. Ideally they should be presented in an integrated fashion, but for purposes of exposition we will treat them separately. It is also incorrect to imagine that assessment can be divided into a fixed sequence of stages; the divisions below have been adopted solely for clarity of presentation and are not meant to imply that assessment can be done according to a 'cookbook' formula. As a final preparatory remark, we must acknowledge that the day of totally objective, precise, behavioural assessment has not yet arrived. Until that day the use of commonsense and careful guesswork will be an important part of assessment, especially in the use of interview techniques (to be discussed below).

In outline, assessment for 'alcoholism' involves four types of inquiry: screening for the existence of alcohol problems, assessments of dependence, cognitive-behavioural problem analyses, goal setting and the monitoring of changes.

Screening for alcohol problems: who is at risk?

Screening is the first and in some respects the most important part of assessment. Most problem drinkers go undetected until far too late, if they are noticed at all. Given the prevalence of alcohol problems and the high miss rate, a wise practice is to suspect a drinking problem whether or not the emotional complaints or behavioural problems patients present have an obvious relation to excessive drinking. Those with alcohol problems are not usually conspicuous as patients and may show up at the clinic with a wide variety of medical or psychiatric problems. Drinking problems may be missed unless their existence is always suspected. In the sphere of psychosocial changes, the following should alert the clinician to enquire about the patient's drinking practices.

(a) *Anxiety* Only a few research papers have looked at drinking problems in patients with major anxiety complaints. All reveal that a substantial proportion drink to excess in misguided attempts to tranquillise their fears.

(b) *Depression* There is no evidence which gives alcohol a causal role in major depressions, but virtually all heavy drinkers suffer from some form of depression. Furthermore, save for the effects of the first few drinks, depression is intensified by the heavy consumption of alcohol. Suicide is a serious risk in the depressed who drink heavily, and the patient's thoughts about suicide must be discussed at the earliest opportunity.

(c) *Violent behaviour* In the interview schedules we reviewed, rarely is violent behaviour mentioned as a sign that serious drinking problems exist. Violence, especially within the family, seems to be considered a phenomenon limited to those who live on the margins of society. That was our belief until we stumbled across the occurrence of violent behaviour within middle-class families we had been seeing for other problems.[3]

The female problem drinker

At this point some comments on women and alcohol are in order because of the idea that problem drinking in women has an altogether different dynamic, takes a different form from male drinking problems and requires different assessment strategies.

In some quarters female alcoholism is held to be a specially malignant form of the disorder. It is argued that if a patient's culture permits heavy drinking then learning factors rather than personality disorders will be of paramount importance in the onset of problem drinking. However, where some or all the population in a culture are censured for heavy drinking then, the argument goes, those who contravene accepted practices do so in the face of opposition, thereby revealing prima facie evidence of an unbalanced personality. The argument is that since there are greater prohibitions against women drinking, once a female drinks regularly to excess she is, perforce, more psychiatrically disturbed than a male who has the same history of excessive drinking. These and related ideas are now coming under attack. Edwards refers to them as the 'lumber of misperception'[4] which has to be removed before women can be treated as individuals and not as exemplars of a homogeneous group afflicted with identical pathologies.

As an example of the traditional thinking consider this extract from a letter of discharge written from the hospital to a woman's family doctor: 'As is usual with these women alcoholics the degree of personality disturbance made treatment difficult'. First, contrary to the flat assertion in the letter, there are no findings proving that female drinkers have a poorer prognosis than males. Nor is there any consistent body of evidence that women ('these women alcoholics') have greater personality disturbances than men. Claims for the existence of such differences when scrutinised closely reveal that all of the adverse correlates for a poor prognosis in women (unmarried, unemployed, with a high degree of alcohol use in their natural parents, poor education) are exactly the same as those which predict a continuation of excessive drinking in men. The differences in personality which distinguish male from female problem drinkers are not ones which have been diagnostic of problem drinking.

The letter goes on to reveal something about the outlook of the therapist: '. . . and I think we have to accept a bad prognosis'. The adverse effects of negative expectancies on clinical outcome have already been covered. They can amount to self-fulfilling prophecies in which failure is expected, predicted and is then blamed on the patient's 'lack of motivation'. To continue the letter: 'Mrs G got little out of the groups and was unwilling to lower her defences and to discuss her neurotic tendencies'. If, as sounds likely, her 'denial' was attacked in a confrontational manner then the results, as we have seen, are unlikely to be favourable. Moreover, when clinicians move away from a discussion of the specifics of the drinking problems (for example, amount consumed, pressure situations, contextual influences, behaviour of family and friends towards drinking) satisfactory outcomes become more rare. The further the therapist directs the discussion away from the presenting problem the greater the risk of failure.

Back to the letter: 'We see her as an inadequate personality with depressive features. With her children grown up, she now has too much time on her hands but does not consider helping her husband in his very busy career. He is a very supportive and long-suffering chap but has clearly had enough and one must sympathise. We have discharged her on [an antidepressant drug]'.[5] There is no mention in this report of what coping techniques and self-control strategies Mrs G can use when drinking pressures arise. Instead she is given her tablets and sent on her way. (Notice too, that there is no Suffering Sam or Controlling Charles mentioned—see Chapter 10.)

Edwards remarks that reports of this sort are common. Often the woman in question is referred to as 'this lass' or 'this girl' and if she is attractive that will feature in the description of her as well. The letter is significant in that it contains the whole network of negative stereotypes about women drinkers. It ends, as Edwards points out, with 'Mrs G being disdained', the disdain being dressed up in professional language.

The growing convergence of the numbers of male and female alcoholics may help to put an end to the belief that while the particulars of each man's case must be studied in careful detail, it is still possible to speculate about women drinkers in a general way.

There are, of course, likely to be differences between male and female problem drinkers. The woman at home is more likely to drink alone, and will probably drink the more affordable wines and sherries that can be managed on the household allowance given by her husband. Because she will have shopping to do and may well have children to look after or fetch from school her drinking is likely to be spread over the day, differing from the archetypal male problem drinker who is inclined to drink more quickly to the point of intoxication. One would expect a less leisurely pattern of consumption in the businesswoman problem drinker, but until the research has been done all of this remains, at best, plausible speculation. The point we wish to stress is that the stereotype of the 'female alcoholic' has been accepted without support.

There are two significant differences between males and females which relate to excessive drinking which are connected to their biologies. For structural and physiological reasons a woman is more at risk of liver damage than a man and, second, as depression is known to cluster with problem drinking the much higher prevalence of depression in women[6] should warn the clinician that an 'innocent' case of depression might conceal a significant alcohol problem.

It should not need saying that the rationale therapies,

courtesies, clinical techniques and self-control methods which have an established record with male drinkers are equally suited to female drinkers. The causes usually cited for female problem drinking (for example, the 'empty nest' syndrome) can be translated into language which establishes parallels with causes that operate in men (for 'empty nest' read 'unemployed and lonely'). A fair reading of the clinical literature on problem drinking females is that the expectations and attitudes have been anything but fair and the time for change is now. In this chapter we will proceed on the assumption that the rules and methods of psychological assessment apply to men and women alike. Clinicians should approach *all* clients with a high 'index of suspicion'.

Screening: tests and techniques

When the clinician's suspicions are roused, further screening steps should be taken. Two of the most popular screening tests are the Michigan Alcoholism Screening Test (MAST)[7] and the CAGE[8] questionnaire. They both have acceptable diagnostic accuracy when compared with laboratory tests.[9]

The CAGE test consists of four questions, the letters of the acronym being the initial letters of a key word in each question:

1. Have you ever felt the need to CUT down on your drinking?
2. Have you felt ANNOYED by others asking you about your drinking?
3. Do you feel GUILTY about your drinking?
4. Do you ever have an EYE-OPENER in the morning?

A score of two 'yes' answers on the CAGE test indicates that drinking problems are likely. The brief MAST has ten items (a longer, 25-item form is also available but is not considered superior) and is designed to give an indication of the severity of drinking problems. A score of 5/10 is suggestive of problem drinking. The questions cover the social, physical and legal costs of drinking. A newer screening device, the Canterbury alcoholism screening test (CAST) has high reliability and very high validation scores, and has the advantage over the CAGE and the MAST of tapping the clinical symptoms of excessive drinking. The full CAST, scoring, validation and reliability data can be found in Appendix A.

The CAGE, MAST, CAST and all other screening tests are not

without their difficulties. The intent of the questions is quite transparent and a respondent who wants to misrepresent his condition can do so easily. Therefore, if the criterion scores are equalled or exceeded it is a safe bet that the patient is experiencing difficulties with alcohol. A low score, on the other hand, is more difficult to interpret. Second, the screening tests are not to be confused with tests of dependence; the CAGE, MAST and CAST, if answered honestly, will detect both dependent and non-dependent drinkers.

At some point early in the proceedings direct estimates of the quantity and frequency of drinking must be obtained. The patient should be asked: 'About how many drinks do you have every day?' (and not 'Do you drink much/often?'). For precision of communication the patient should be introduced to the concept of the 'standard drink'. That is the drink which contains 17.4 ml (or 13.6 g or .60 oz) of ethanol. (In the US 14 ml defines a standard drink.) In Australia and North America most full strength beers contain approximately 5 per cent absolute alcohol by volume. Table wines are in the vicinity of 10 to 15 per cent absolute alcohol, while fortified wines, such as port and vermouth, contain 20 per cent or slightly less. For distilled spirits (whisky, vodka) the figure is about 40 per cent. Definitions of a standard drink (using the criteria of the Addiction Research Foundation of Ontario) which are in use in North America are:

340 ml (about 12 oz) of regular beer
140 ml (about 5 oz) of table wine
85 ml (about 3 oz) of fortified wine
43 ml (about 1.5 oz) of spirits.

In Australia standard drinks are defined as follows:

425 ml (15 oz) of low alcohol beer
285 ml (10 oz) of regular beer
120 ml (4 oz) of table wine
60 ml (2 oz) of fortified wine
30 ml (1 oz) of spirits.

'How much is too much?' depends on whether one is asking the question from a legal or a health standpoint. If legal limits for driving are the concern, a blood alcohol level over .05 (or whatever) is too much. A wide range of serious physical disorders is predicted if consumption passes six standard drinks each day for men (four for women). Four drinks each day (three for women) can bring about a significant risk of liver cirrhosis.[10] The previous data all refer to the correlation between drinking levels and medical problems. There is evidence that adverse social and psychological consequences are associated with even lower levels of consumption. Sanchez-Craig's recent study[11] sought an empirically derived criterion of consumption that divided problem from problem-free drinking. The criterion arrived at was four or more drinks three days a week. Five and a half drinks on four days a week was clearly correlated with self-identified problem drinking (for example, complaints of sleep problems, reported difficulties with coping with negative emotions and the presence of inter-personal conflicts), although which is cause and which is effect cannot be told from this correlation.

When asking for an estimate of the number of drinks each day, a drinking diary can be used, but underestimates are fairly likely. A way sometimes used to elicit more accurate estimates of average intake is known as the 'top-high' technique. It has been found that if different groups of drinkers are given numbers to circle to indicate the number of drinks they have had each day, the sheet which has the larger range of figures printed on it will elicit higher results. As an example, if a sheet asks '1, 2, 3, 4, 5, 6 or more (please specify)' lower estimates will be made than if the sheet offers categories in the higher ranges: '1, 2, 3, 4, 5, 6, 7, 8, 9, 10 or more (please specify)'.

If screening questions uncover the existence of alcohol problems, the next step is to obtain a drinking history. Asking the patient to retrieve memories of long-past periods of his life is unlikely to yield an exact pattern of drinking or an accurate life history. A discussion of the rationale for the format for a general history taking is not within the scope of our current aims, but a take-home life-history questionnaire can be found in Lazarus' book *Behaviour Therapy and Beyond.*[12] Questionnaires cover the basic areas in which information needs to be gathered and save valuable clinical time. The open-ended questions give the patients the opportunity to list troubling matters which they may find too difficult to broach initially in a face-to-face discussion. The purpose of a general drinking history is to give a longitudinal perspective on the patient's problems with alcohol and a context for the investigation of current drinking behaviour and its meaning for the patient.

It is rare to find in the course of the history that the patient's alcohol problems have risen to and have thereafter remained at a high and steady state. The pattern to be expected will be dynamic and not static.[13] The patient may never have paid attention to these changes or the patterns they form in relation to life events. Both belong in an outline of drinking history.

The questions that follow help to give that perspective.

1. When did you have your first drink?
2. How old were you when you began to drink regularly?
3. When did you first have spirits to drink?
4. When did you begin to drink each day?
5. When did heavy drinking begin? How old were you? Were you still at school or were you working?
6. If you ever attempted to give up drinking, when did you make your first (second, etc.) attempt? How long did it last? Why did you try to give it up (or try to cut down)? Did you have any help (friends, spouse, AA)?
7. When did drinking first seem to be a problem to you?
8. When did your drinking first seem to be a problem to others?
9. Where did the troubles show up first (in your social life, your work, your marriage, your health)?
10. Which concerned you most?
11. Do you think your drinking is a problem now?
12. In what ways (for example, effects on health, work performance, marital life, other)?
13. At the start of regular drinking, where and with whom did you drink? Is that still the case or has it changed?
14. What were your main reasons for drinking at the time when it began to change from regular drinking to problem drinking (for example, for pleasure, just going along with others, helping you to forget your worries and the fact that you were feeling down)?
15. What are the main reasons now?
16. How much and how often did you drink when:
    (a) you left school?
    (b) you left home?
    (c) you got married or had your first permanent relationship?
    (d) you got your first job?

(e) (and if) you lost a job?
(f) (and if) a significant relationship broke up?

17. Describe a recent day (within the last three months) when, in your view, your drinking was heavy.
18. At what point, on that day, did your drinking seem to become too much? Why do you think you kept on drinking past that point?
19. Describe a typical drinking day. How much do you drink over what period of time?
20. Why do you continue to drink (to relieve distress, physical or emotional; because your friends or people you spend time with do; other)?
21. How many drinks does it take to make you feel
    (a) 'high' but without seeming or feeling drunk?
    (b) drunk (for example, having trouble in speaking clearly)?
22. What would you estimate your drinking pattern to be over the last three months:

Quantity	Number of days
0	
1–3	
4–7	
7–10	
10–13	
13–16	
16+	

23. Of the people who live with you, how many:
    (a) drink more than you do?
    (b) drink the same amount as you do?
    (c) drink less than you do?
24. Of those outside the family (friends, people you work with) who drink with you, how many:
    (a) drink more than you do?
    (b) drink the same amount as you do?
    (c) drink less than you do?
25. Are there any people living with you who are likely to put pressure on you to drink, even if they know that your goal is not to drink more, or at all? Friends? Workmates?

26. Do you ever take a few drinks or more, on your own, when you are drinking with others?
27. Do you drink mostly
    (a) beer?
    (b) wine?
    (c) spirits?
    (d) all of the above?
    (e) mixed drinks?
    (f) other drinks (please specify)?
28. Do you ever drink before breakfast? If so, how often?

Questions 1 to 20 are designed to assess the existence, and especially the drinker's awareness, of problems with alcohol over a lifetime, with a focus on a recent and representative time. Question 21 is a 'tolerance' question, while 22 is aimed at quantity-frequency measures. Questions 23, 24 and 25 ask about the models in the drinker's social environment and whether he is likely to be subjected to pressure to continue with his hazardous drinking. Questions 26 and 28, which are answered in the affirmative by those with more serious drinking problems, suggest the need for a careful assessment of dependence (to be discussed later in this chapter).

The questionnaire is a supplement to the screening assessment but is not the same as the self-recording diary technique, in which a diary is filled in every day and reviewed at each meeting, and which is closely tied to clinical intervention.

Controlled drinking or total abstinence?

The literature reviewed in the preceding chapters requires us to discard the concept of alcoholism as a single disorder requiring a single treatment. Some forms of controlled drinking are helpful, even necessary, for certain problem drinkers while other drinkers can only recover if they keep to a decision of abstinence. For yet others the matter may have to be negotiated in the light of on-going results. The decision will depend upon a number of considerations:

Physical health

If there is any evidence of a physical infirmity, such as severe liver damage, diabetes or other potentially lethal disabilities which might eventuate were the patient to drink at all, then the therapist must urge total abstinence.

Affective disorders

The link between affective disorders, especially depression, and drinking is strong. Weissman et al.[14] tested a large American population and found that among the group diagnosed as alcoholic 70 per cent had at one time or another in their lives received at least one or more psychiatric diagnoses, the most frequent being depression. The depression was considered 'primary' and not the ubiquitous dysphoria-depression caused by chronic intoxication. What happens to depressives who drink? Mayfield puts it concisely: 'If you feel very bad alcohol will make you feel a lot better. But if you drink a lot of alcohol it will make you feel very bad';[15] 'chronic intoxication is regularly accompanied by affective discomfort that is progressive as intoxication continues. This deterioration in affective state has been observed to proceed to the point of a severe depressive syndrome with suicidal ideation. With cessation of drinking this [severe] mood disturbance promptly disappears.' The irresistible inference to be drawn from the potentially deadly connection between alcohol and depression is the need to strongly recommend total abstinence, regardless of dependence levels, at least until depression has been brought under control.

Schizophrenia

It was not until 1965,[16] with the publication of Pokorny's work on the problems of alcohol abuse in psychiatric patients that clinicians took note of the complications of excessive drinking in schizophrenic individuals. There are no good studies, or much of a literature at all, on treatment outcomes with schizophrenics who drink to excess. That they do so in sufficient numbers for a study to be carried out is likely; one study found that 15 per cent of a diagnosed schizophrenic population were excessive drinkers. It has also been discovered that there are a number of negative consequences in schizophrenics associated with alcohol abuse (mood deterioration, behaviour problems, hallucinations, seizures, diabetes and peripheral neuropathy). These reactions, plus the potential for adverse cross reactions between alcohol and the major tranquillisers in universal use with schizophrenics, strongly suggest that the most sensible course for any patient with a history of schizophrenia is to avoid alcohol altogether. Will schizophrenics in remission or those who are actively psychotic take advice along these lines? These questions have been considered in only the most preliminary fashion, but the few results that are available seem to indicate that they will.[17]

Levels of dependence

In Chapter 3 we looked at the notion of dependence and its relevance to theoretical controversies still being fought out in the field of alcohol studies. The position taken there, and throughout the book, borrows from the ideas of Griffith Edwards on the issue: 'Dependence is a highly important clinical reality and an understanding of all its implications is one essential part of the therapist's competence if he is to deal with drinking problems. But nothing which is being said should be misinterpreted as implying that dependence is everything. Dependence only exists in a personal and social context and it would be an absurd abstraction ever to see things otherwise. Furthermore, and as has already been stressed, many patients with drinking problems are not suffering from the dependence syndrome'.[18] In other words, measures of dependence, if they could always be gathered with high predictive validity, and they cannot, would still not constitute a clinical 'magic bullet' for uncomplicated assessment.

In very broad terms dependence is taken to mean impaired control over drinking (but not some kind of biochemical chain reaction leading automatically to 'loss of control'), increased tolerance, subjective 'craving' and an array of withdrawal reactions which make their appearance when the usual period of time between drinking elapses without any or the usual intake of alcohol. Severely dependent drinkers are likely either to be abstinent or drinking to great excess. With such people there is a much reduced likelihood of controlled drinking: 'the presence of alcohol dependence symptoms (for example, tremulousness, morning drinking, blackouts) even at very low levels is a serious indication and is predictive of continuing alcohol problems in the future'.[19] The reservations of Shaw[20] are well taken but increasingly cognitive-behaviourist therapists are prepared to view controlled drinking options with serious reservations in drinkers who display significant levels of dependence.

For the practicing clinician the starting point is obtaining reliable measures of dependence which have obtained unchallenged acceptance. Unfortunately there is no one universally recognised test or set of questions for this purpose. A number of pencil and paper tests are in use and readily available. The Alcohol Dependence Scale (ADS)[21] is a 25-item self-report questionnaire. The questions are of the 'imagine if' variety (for example, the person is asked to imagine that he has been completely abstaining from alcohol for a few days and then drinking heavily for a few days. He is then asked to indicate how he would feel on the morning after). An 0 score gives no evidence of dependence (reported); 1–13 suggest a low level of dependence, in which case the patient is more likely to comply with controlled drinking goals; 14–21 are in the moderate range and controlled drinking may be considered; 22–30 indicate a substantial level of alcohol dependence and abstinence goals should seriously be considered; and 31–47 are rated as severe dependence and abstinence is really the only reasonable treatment goal. The ADS scale is favoured with good validity data, reported in a 1982 paper:[22]

(a) *Compliance* Those who scored in the lowest range were most likely to keep their appointments; those in the highest range of scores (31–47) were least likely to keep their first treatment appointments.

(b) *Consumption and psychological and physical problems* Higher scores on the ADS were correlated with higher levels of consumption and a variety of problems ranging from social and occupational instability, to thought disorders and physical symptoms, most notably a marked prevalence of digestive disorders (linked to liver disease).

(c) *Patient expectancies about controlled drinking* When patients were asked if they believed that they could cut down their drinking to a moderate level the majority answered in the affirmative; at the highest level on the ADS, 89 per cent believed that abstinence was the only way that they could improve.

The second of the two best known tests of dependence, the SADQ[23], has already been mentioned. This instrument contains 20 questions, each of which can be answered in one of four categories: 'almost never', 'sometimes', 'often' and 'nearly always', scored 0, 1, 2 and 3 respectively. The questions are heavily weighted toward the assessment of physical dependence and neuroadaptive changes to chronic drinking, particularly on withdrawal reactions the morning after a day of heavy drinking. The SADQ, then, has a biological emphasis (which more cognitively oriented writers see as a flaw). To illustrate, here are two examples: 'During a heavy drinking period, I wake up feeling sweaty'; 'During a heavy drinking period my hands shake first thing in the morning'. It is customary to rate those who score above 30, out of a possible 60, as highly dependent and for the clinician to give patients who score in this range no encouragement to believe that they can ever again drink alcohol safely.

In 1986 validity data on a Short Alcohol Dependence Data (SADD) questionnaire were reported.[24] The 15-item test correlated highly with the SADQ but was rather better than the latter in discriminating between individuals in the mild to moderate range. The recent development of the SADD means that it has yet to be tested thoroughly, but it has the advantage of conceptualising dependence as a clustering of cognitive, behavioural and physiological reactions. The authors stress the importance of detecting alcohol problems in patients who develop chronic alcohol-related diseases of the liver. The SADD was constructed with the whole of the drinking population in mind, and attempts to tap cognitive and behavioural reactions to the excessive use of alcohol.

Finally, Heather, Rollnick and Winton[25] used a 'subjective' estimate carried out via 10 questions (for example, 'At the present time, after drinking one drink, could you stop if you wanted to?'; 'At the present time do you believe that you have, or could have, control over your drinking, that is, could you drink socially?') They compared their subjective test with the 'objective' SADQ in a group of male and female alcoholics who had been treated for abstinence in an alcohol unit. At six-month follow-up the 'subjective' test but not the SADQ significantly predicted those who returned to harmful drinking. The results provided support for a two-stage model of relapse: one, does the person remain abstinent? And two, if he has a drink, does he return to harmful levels of drinking? The authors' conclusions on the superiority of their test over the SADQ, given that the SADQ is the leading assessment device in terms of experimental and clinical investigation, are that it is 'all the more remarkable when it is remembered that it was very much an ad hoc instrument . . . One explanation for [its superiority] might be that the SADQ is itself a poor measuring instrument, despite the evidence of high internal consistency against a clinician's ratings of severity of dependence. It is more likely, however . . . that the alcoholic patient's cognitive interpretation of his dependence on alcohol, which is heavily influenced by the understandings of alcohol dependence to which he has been exposed, is more important than the psychobiological phenomena in determining the probability of relapse.'[26] Heather and his colleagues take care not to dismiss the importance of dependence, or the role of psychobiological changes in it, but they also hold to the view that 'cognitive factors'—the patient's interpretation of his behaviour vis a vis alcohol—are more important still.

These words are well taken. There is a risk that the clinician, in an attempt to make sense of the bewildering collection of problems and possibilities confronting him may be tempted to turn to one of the available assessment devices just mentioned and use it as though it were some kind of psychological x-ray supplying an unambiguous and error-free measure of a 'dependence disorder'. To believe that would be to miss the reasons for discarding the disease concept of alcoholism in the first place. Drinking alcohol is an activity, something that a person does, and not a thing that he 'has'. The clinician must be on guard against using dependence as a new word for alcoholism. Hodgson and Edwards, who make extensive use of the dependence construct, take care to caution against turning to dependence as a panacea notion which will permit the clinician to ignore the role in the treatment plan of the patient's contributions, his interpretation of his drinking, how it affects him, his skills and the social supports available to him. Drinking and excessive drinking occur in response to a complex of learned psychosocial cues and psychobiological urges. If there is one idea which captures the problem of dependence from the drinker's point of view it is not the frequent or excessive use of alcohol but the amount of difficulty in refraining from the further intake of alcohol on a given occasion.

How clinically useful are the dependence scales now in use? The alcohol dependence syndrome construct was derived from careful and sustained clinical observation. While questionnaires may attempt to assess this construct, no questionnaire can replace the integrative and intuitive capacity of the experienced clinician.

Cognitive abilities and neuropsychological functioning

People with histories of prolonged excessive drinking demonstrate significantly greater impairments in cognitive (intellectual) functioning than control groups of moderate drinkers or life-long abstainers.[27] Performance deficiencies have been equated with a variety of cerebral dysfunctions. There is evidence for alcohol-induced damage to a number of brain structures (both cerebral hemispheres, the limbic system and the parietal lobe areas have all been proposed as crucial sites) which has been cited to account for the cognitive deficits associated with long-term drinking. Recent interpretations favour the conclusion that the disorder is diffuse and not restricted to one specific system. The neuropsychological research available which is related to treatment outcome indicates that the major areas of psychological functioning impaired by excessive drinking are the abilities to abstract, to learn new information and to solve problems. Given that current approaches to treatment emphasise learning new coping strategies and more adaptive problem-solving skills (highly-practiced skills, general knowledge and language abilities are left relatively intact), cognitive deficits could prove a serious barrier to the acquisition of new skills and strategies upon which cognitive-behavioural therapies are based. The brighter side is that neuropsychological status, whatever its connection to specific brain systems, can improve significantly with as little as 15 to 30 days of sobriety. In a 1981 study of problem drinkers, Wilkinson and Sanchez-Craig found that socially stable patients showed significantly more improvement following three weeks of abstinence if they drank one drink or nothing each day, than a similar group who drank, on average, four drinks per day (although the four-drink amount was well below their pretreatment levels). Unless future studies contradict the evidence now available, patients who show cognitive deficits (as measured by cognitive tests like the Digit Symbol of the WAIS and the Raven Matrices) should be counselled to abstain from drinking any alcohol, or to drink very little.

Social support and social stability

The availability of a network of social support is a major asset. Patients who are married and have job and residential stability will fare better in any treatment programme, regardless of the interventions employed or the goals adopted, than those without such forms of social stability. There is reason to believe that married drinkers may do better with abstinence rather than controlled drinking goals. The difficulty in interpreting this evidence is that married drinkers are usually older, are likely to have a longer drinking history[28] and are possibly more dependent. But whatever the correct interpretation of the uncontrolled studies mentioned, it is necessary to canvass feelings amongst significant others before arriving at a final decision (contraindications absent). Our experience, in accord with others, is that if the spouse or others close to the drinker strongly believe that abstinence is the correct solution it is unlikely that moderate drinking goals will be achieved.

Duration of problem drinking

The best available data make moderation seem the more reasonable objective, all things being equal, if problem drinking has been of a fairly short duration. 'Problem' as used here refers to the time since drinking began to cause difficulties in the drinker's job performance, social life or general well-being. The clinical findings suggest that successful controlled drinkers are more often found to be younger drinkers (under 40 years of age). It could be that because they are less likely to subscribe to the alcoholic stereotype ('one drink, one drunk'). They tend to give a different meaning to their episodes of excessive drinking than do older drinkers, who are more ready to accept the designation 'alcoholic' and all that it implies. An equally plausible explanation is that older problem drinkers have consumed more alcohol and as a result have climbed to higher levels of dependence.

To summarise, it is now acepted that problem drinkers/alcoholics make up a diverse group. Clinical observations and experimental studies reveal that the diversities can be grouped into two broad areas: the origins of the drinking problem and the varieties of difficulties it causes, or exacerbates. It is true that there is more to drinking problems than drinking itself, but the direct and indirect costs of taking too much alcohol, too often, make the modification of the consumption the immediate focus and the most vital concern of assessment and therapy. Judgements about the pace and extent of modification are a complex function of dependence levels, drinking history, coexisting psychological and physiological complaints and not least of all the drinker's faith in change and his motivation to take the difficult steps involved in changing his drinking, and his life.

CHAPTER 7

Medical Aspects of Management: Basic Pharmacology of Alcohol and Principles of Assessment

John B. Saunders

Introduction

Alcohol-related problems are commonly seen in medical practice. Indeed, doctors probably see more problem drinkers than any other health professional group. There is unfortunately a tendency for doctors to concentrate on treating the presenting syndrome, be it physical or neuropsychiatric, at the expense of the underlying drinking problem. However, the availability of medical skills is important for a high proportion of persons with drinking problems. Medical therapy for withdrawal states and the physical and neuropsychiatric complications may be lifesaving. It is important for all therapists to know the scope of medical management and the range of investigations and treatments available.

Before the presenting features of alcohol-related problems and the principles and practice of medical assessment are described, an account is given of the pharmacology of alcohol. Therapists are frequently asked for advice on the effects of alcohol and on safe drinking practices. It is necessary to have sufficient knowledge of the way in which alcohol is handled by the body and the pharmacological effects of alcohol to provide a considered opinion.

The Pharmacology of Alcohol

Absorption, distribution and elimination

Alcohol is a simple chemical substance with a molecular weight of 46. It is absorbed rapidly from the gastrointestinal tract, principally from the upper small bowel (80 per cent) and to a lesser extent from the stomach (20 per cent). It then enters the systemic circulation, via the liver, and the peak blood alcohol concentration is reached 30 to 60 minutes after a single dose. Because of its solubility characteristics, alcohol distributes into the 'lean body mass' (which includes the brain, muscles, liver and other internal organs) but only to a limited extent into fatty tissue or bone. The volume of distribution for alcohol is lower in women than in men because women have proportionately more fat and a smaller lean body mass. Consequently, blood alcohol concentrations are, on average, higher in women than in men after an equivalent dose, as shown in Fig. 7.1.

Alcohol is eliminated from the body predominantly by oxidative metabolism. The liver is the main site of metabolism, accounting for 90 to 95 per cent of the amount taken; 3 to 5 per cent is metabolised elsewhere. Urinary excretion and exhalation in breath account for about 2 to 3 per cent each. Metabolism

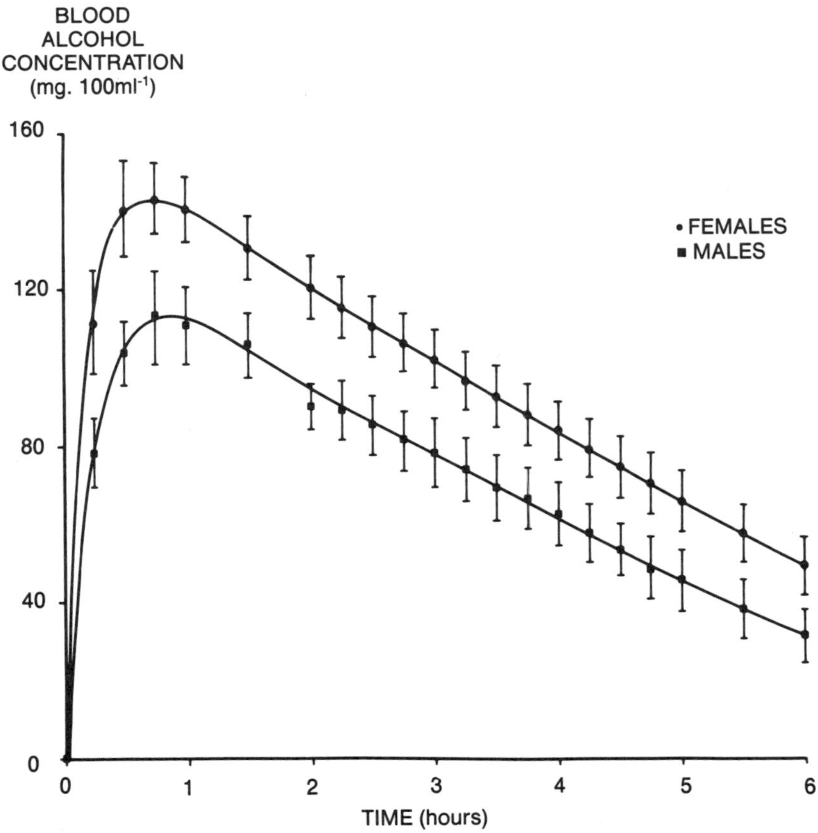

Figure 7.1 Blood alcohol concentrations after an oral dose in healthy subjects.

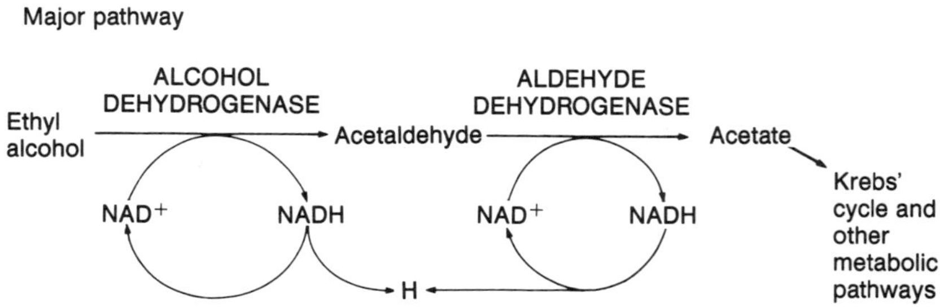

Figure 7.2 Metabolism of alcohol.

involves a two-stage oxidation, as shown in Fig. 7.2. The first step is conversion to acetaldehyde via the enzyme alcohol dehydrogenase. Acetaldehyde is a toxic and chemically reactive substance. Normally it is rapidly metabolised, via the enzyme aldehyde dehydrogenase, to acetate which is further metabolised, ultimately to carbon dioxide and water. Hydrogen equivalents produced in the first two stages fuel several subsidiary reactions which result *inter alia* in production of fats, lactic acid and uric acid. The average rate of elimination of alcohol from blood is 15 mg/100 ml/hr (0.015 g/100 ml/hr), which is equivalent to 10 g (or one standard drink) per hour for a 70 kg person. A deficiency of aldehyde dehydrogenase is found in approximately 50 per cent of persons of oriental (mongoloid) race, such as Chinese and Japanese. In persons with this enzyme deficiency alcohol causes an acute flushing reaction affecting the face and upper trunk. This is caused by accumulation of acetaldehyde.

The blood alcohol concentration reached after drinking depends not only on the amount taken but also on:

1. *The time over which drinks are consumed* The blood alcohol concentration will be lower if drinking takes place over several hours than if the same amount is consumed over a shorter period.
2. *The interval since the last drink* The blood alcohol concentration may not have returned to zero.
3. *The type of drink consumed* Alcohol is absorbed most rapidly as a 20 per cent solution, for example vermouth, or spirits diluted with water or tonic, compared with beer or undiluted spirits.

4. *Whether alcohol is taken on an empty stomach or after a meal* The presence of food in the stomach retards the absorption of alcohol and results in lower average blood alcohol concentrations.
5. *Body weight and composition* Blood alcohol concentrations are lower in muscular than in fat persons of the same weight.
6. *Sex* See Figure 7.1.
7. *The rate of alcohol metabolism* This shows considerable variation from person to person. This is partly explained on a genetic basis.
8. *Previous alcohol and drug intake* Chronic consumption of alcohol and certain drugs increases the rate of alcohol metabolism and can result in lower blood alcohol concentrations. On the other hand some drugs inhibit alcohol metabolism and result in higher concentrations sustained for longer.
9. *Concurrent disease* Chronic liver disease decreases the rate of alcohol metabolism. Gastric surgery may increase the rate of absorption.

Because of these factors it is impossible to predict accurately the blood alcohol concentration that will occur at any particular time after drinking. As a very rough guide, three standard drinks taken over 30 minutes will result in a peak blood alcohol concentration of approximately 50 mg/100 ml (0.05 g/100 ml) one hour after the last drink and five to six standard drinks will result in a blood alcohol concentration approaching 100 mg/100 ml (0.10 g/100 ml).

Acute effects of alcohol

The most obvious acute effects are those on the central nervous system (CNS). Alcohol is a non-specific CNS depressant and has many actions in common with sedative-hypnotic drugs. This might seem surprising as the initial effects of alcohol (talkativeness and increased self-confidence) appear to be stimulatory. This is explained by the fact that at low blood alcohol concentrations there is proportionately greater inhibition of higher centres, which themselves inhibit certain behaviours.

The symptoms experienced after drinking depend on:

(a) the blood alcohol concentration;
(b) the tolerance to alcohol that has developed;

(c) whether the blood alcohol concentration is rising or falling; and
(d) whether there is a deficiency in aldehyde dehydrogenase (which results in the idiosyncratic flushing reaction).

Broadly there are two types of effect—on behaviour and on psychomotor function and coordination. In non-tolerant drinkers, altered behaviour and changes in psychomotor performance are discernable at blood alcohol concentrations of only 30 mg/100 ml (0.03 g/100 ml). Typically the drinker feels more relaxed and is more talkative. There is impairment of judgement. As the blood alcohol concentration rises further there is usually a feeling of euphoria and disinhibition. If drinking continues this is followed by emotional lability and then, successively, by apathy and drowsiness. Performance of complex tasks (especially multiple or simultaneous ones) worsens with each increment in the blood alcohol concentration over 30 mg/100 ml. At 50 mg/100 ml (0.05 g/100 ml) there is a significantly increased risk of an accident. The risk is two-fold for having a road traffic accident when driving at this level. Coordination becomes progressively impaired so that at a blood alcohol concentration of 200 mg/100 ml (0.20 g/100 ml), a non-tolerant drinker is usually unable to stand or walk. When the blood alcohol concentration exceeds 300 mg/100 ml (0.30 g/100 ml) the person is usually comatose and may die from respiratory depression.

The effects listed in Table 7.1 occur in tolerant drinkers at proportionately higher blood alcohol concentrations. Tolerance is likely to develop in persons who regularly drink more than 60 g alcohol (six standard drinks) per day and is an integral feature of the alcohol dependence syndrome. The effects listed in Table 7.1 may not be manifest until the blood alcohol concentration is three to four times higher than is indicated there. However, the degree of tolerance that develops to the anaesthetising effects of alcohol and the depressant effects on the vital centres in the brain which subserve respiration and cardiovascular function, is much less. As a result, the lethal concentration may be little higher in the tolerant drinker than in the novice.

The pleasant effects of alcohol, such as a feeling of wellbeing and relaxation, are typically experienced when the blood alcohol concentration is rising shortly after drinking has commenced.

TABLE 7.1
Effects of Alcohol at Various Blood Alcohol Concentrations

Blood alcohol concentration (BAC) mg/100ml	(g%)	Likely effects (during upswing of BAC curve)
30	0.03	Feeling of well-being and relaxation. More talkative. Slightly slower reactions.
50	0.05	Euphoria. Increased self-confidence. Impairment of attention, judgement and psychomotor reactions. Increased risk of accidents.
75	0.075	Disinhibition. Garrulousness. Further loss of judgement and coordination. Nausea.
100	0.10	Emotional instability. Argumentativeness. Impaired balance. Onset of ataxia (staggering gait). Slurred speech. Dizziness. Desire to sleep when not in company.
150	0.15	Confusion and disorientation. Apathy. Drowsiness and sleep. Decreased pain sensation. Worsening ataxia.
200	0.20	Stupor. Inertia. Inability to stand or walk. Vomiting. Incontinence.
300+	0.30+	Coma. Anaesthesia. Hypothermia. Possible death from respiratory paralysis, aspiration of vomit.

Note that the effects are typical of those experienced by non-tolerant drinkers. When tolerance has developed the effects on behaviour and coordination may not be seen until the blood alcohol concentration is three to four times higher. Note also that dysphoria, apathy and nausea are commonly experienced at blood alcohol concentrations below 75 mg/100 ml during the downswing of the BAC curve.

When the blood alcohol concentration has returned to the same level from a higher one, the predominant feelings may be of dysphoria, apathy, uneasiness and nausea.

In addition to the effects on the CNS, alcohol has a multiplicity of effects on other parts of the body. These will not be discussed further but the reader is referred to a comprehensive review by Lieber.[1]

The range of presenting problems

At the outset it should be emphasised that only a small minority of patients with a drinking problem spontaneously mention this when attending for medical help. An important role for the doctor is that of detective, for the physical, psychological and social consequences of alcohol consumption are innumerable (Table 7.2) and result in a constellation of clinical syndromes that are remarkable for their diversity. Frequently, the initial complaints are non-specific. Common reasons why patients seek help include 'nerves', anxiety, sleep disturbance, depression, sexual dysfunction, dyspepsia, anorexia, vomiting, recurrent headaches or muscle cramps, to name but a few. In many instances the suspicion that a person has a drinking problem is aroused because of its effect on the family. Perhaps the children look unhappy and uncared for or the long-suffering wife (or husband) is constantly attending with non-specific physical or nervous complaints. Sometimes the harmful drinking is obvious but more likely, at least in the early stages, it is not, and it may take considerable effort by the clinician to establish that alcohol is the fundamental problem.

Detection of problem drinking

It will be apparent that the problem drinker can easily be missed and that correct diagnosis and effective management may be delayed considerably. It is appropriate to consider some ways in which prompt diagnosis can be effected.

High index of suspicion

Given the protean manifestations of harmful drinking and the high prevalence of the problem, it is not overstating the case to say that the clinician should consider this possibility in the majority of patients seen. There is no substitute for the alert clinician with a high index of suspicion.

Key indicators

Virtually none of the problems listed in Table 7.2 is specific to alcohol. Most have other causes and there are relatively few pathognomonic symptoms, clinical signs or laboratory findings. These features, non-specific individually, gain greater significance if they occur together and there are certain combinations

TABLE 7.2
Alcohol-related Problems

PHYSICAL

Intoxication
- Stupor
- Ataxia
- Coma
- Respiratory depression
- Inhalation of vomit and asphyxiation

Liver Disease
- Fatty Liver
- Alcoholic hepatitis
- Cirrhosis

Gastrointestinal diseases
- Carcinoma of oropharynx
- Reflux oesophagitis
- Gastritis
- Malabsorption
- Acute pancreatitis
- Chronic pancreatitis

Brain Damage
- Wernicke-Korsakoff syndrome
- Frontal Lobe syndrome
- Cerebellar disease
- Central pontine myelinolysis
- Subdural haematoma
- Hypertensive stroke

Other neurological diseases
- Optic neuropathy
- Myelopathy
- Peripheral neuropathy
- Autonomic neuropathy

Cardiovascular diseases
- Cardiomyopathy
- Alcohol-induced arrhythmias
- Hypertension

Respiratory diseases
- Aspiration pneumonia
- Upper lobe pneumococcal pneumonia
- Pulmonary tuberculosis

Endocrine and metabolic disorders
- Hypothalmic-pituitary dysfunction
- Testicular atrophy
- Impotence
- Hypoglycaemia
- Pseudo-Cushing's syndrome
- Lactic acidosis
- Gout

Musculoskeletal disorders
- Acute rhabdomyolysis
- Acute myopathy
- Chronic myopathy
- Osteoporosis
- Avascular necrosis of hip
- Gout

Trauma
- Head injury
- Subdural haematoma
- Fractures of rib
- Fractures of long bones
- Multiple trauma (from road accidents etc.)

Fetus
- Fetal alcohol syndrome
- Low birth weight
- Second trimester abortion

Nutritional disturbance
- Protein-caloric malnutrition
- Wernicke-Korsakoff syndrome
- Beri-beri
- Pellagra
- Scurvy
- Zinc deficiency
- Night blindness (vitamin A deficiency)

PSYCHOLOGICAL

Features of dependence and withdrawal
- Compulsion to drink alcohol
- Anxiety and agitation
- Malaise and lethargy
- Depression
- Confusion
- Disorientation
- Hallucination
- Paranoia

Other disturbances
- Anxiety states
- Phobic disorders
- Panic attacks
- Reactive depression
- Amnesic episodes (alcoholic 'blackouts')
  - 'en bloc'
  - fragmentary
- 'Pathological intoxication'
- Transient hallucinatory experience
- Acute alcoholic hallucinosis
- Chronic delusional psychosis ('alcoholic paranoia')
- Deterioration in moral and ethical standards
- Self-centredness
- Inability to cope
- Suicidal ideation
- Suicidal attempt

SOCIAL

Domestic and allied problems
- Loss of friends
- Deterioration in marital and other significant relationships
- Separation
- Divorce

Occupational
- Failure to gain promotion
- Demotion
- Dismissal
- Unemployment

Financial problems
- Loss of regular income from employment
- Hardship from money spent on alcohol
- Gambling debts
- Victim of fraud

Legal Problems
- Drink-driving offences
- Loss of motor vehicle licence
- Property crime
- Assault
- Homicide
- Neglect of children

Miscellaneous
- Prostitution

that are highly suggestive of harmful alcohol consumption. For example, the recently divorced 42-year-old man with hypertension who complains of difficulty sleeping and who has a history of frequent bouts of 'gastric upset', particularly on Mondays, is a prime suspect. An ability to recognise clusters of seemingly unrelated problems from the physical, psychological and social spheres is the hallmark of the successful diagnostician. Some useful 'early indicators' are listed in Table 7.3.

Systematic drinking history

A systematic drinking history should be taken in every patient. It

TABLE 7.3
Early Indicators of Hazardous and Harmful Alcohol Consumption

HAZARDOUS ALCOHOL CONSUMPTION

Alcohol Intake
- Regular drinking of more than 60 g alcohol per day (males) or 40 g per day (females)
- Episodes of intoxication twice monthly or more

Drinking behaviour (including early dependence)
- Gulping the first drinks
- Difficulty in stopping drinking once started
- Most leisure activities involve drinking
- Most friends are heavy drinkers
- Eating lightly or skipping meals while drinking
- Attempts to cut down on drinking which have had limited success

HARMFUL ALCOHOL CONSUMPTION

Psychosocial problems
- Amnesic episodes while intoxicated ('blackouts')
- Insomnia and nightmares
- Accidents in which alcohol is involved
- Charges of 'driving under the influence'
- Lateness or absence from work
- Concern or worry about drinking by self and/or family

Physical symptoms
- Dyspepsia
- Morning nausea and vomiting
- Recurrent diarrhoea

General appearance
- Bloated facies (may be Cushingoid)
- Facial telangiectasia
- Conjunctival injection
- Coating of tongue
- Scars and bruises (especially of varying age)

Demeanour
- Anxious and agitated

Cardiovascular signs
- Tachycardia
- Hypertension

Abdominal signs
- Soft hepatomegaly

Trauma
- Rib fractures

should include an enquiry about the level and frequency of alcohol consumption, about symptoms of alcohol dependence and of problems relating to drinking. The timing of the drinking history within the interview depends on whether any clues to harmful drinking have been elicited, on the nature of the presenting problem and also on the clinician's particular approach to interviewing.

Collateral information

A history of the patient's alcohol consumption, dependence and problems should be elicited from the spouse, another relative or friend. It is usually wise to seek consent from the patient first, depending on the particular circumstances. Collateral information is especially necessary in patients who exhibit strong denial of their alcohol problem. Important information can also be obtained from the hospital medical record or that of the family physician. Such sources are neglected to a surprising degree.

The background to drinking

In tracing the development of the alcohol problem, clues to its genesis may be revealed from the major landmarks in the patient's life, the family dynamics and the occurrence of psychiatric disorders. Many factors are associated with a predisposition to harmful drinking and alcohol dependence, and although a full discussion is outside the scope of this chapter, a brief commentary on some of the more important ones is presented.

Ethnic and cultural background

The drinking practices of peoples from different countries and cultures show great variation and in countries where there is great cultural diversity such as the USA and Australia many different styles of drinking are represented. Among older, first-generation migrants the traditional pattern of drinking tends to be maintained but in the younger age groups and especially in the second and subsequent generations, it is more usually supplemented by that of the indigenous peer group. Although systematic data are lacking, it seems that harmful drinking is more common in Portuguese, Yugoslav, Polish and Finnish migrants than in the general population. Complications of unremitting daily drinking such as cirrhosis are particularly common in migrants from southern

Europe where this pattern of drinking is characteristic, whereas problems arising from binge drinking are more likely to occur in those from Poland and Finland, for a similar reason. The incidence of harmful drinking is especially high amongst Aboriginal people in Australia and American Indians in the USA and its consequences are very severe. Alcohol-related trauma from motor vehicle accidents and violence is a major cause of morbidity and mortality in young people from these ethnic groups.

Family history

There is evidence for a genetic influence on normal and abnormal drinking behaviour. In some families the degree of familial aggregation is very marked, to the extent that a majority of the male members have a drinking problem. A highly heritable 'subtype' of alcoholism has been described.

More important reasons for the familial association are the modelling of drinking behaviour on that of older members of the family and pathological family dynamics.

Personality traits and personality disorders

The concept of a specific personality trait that predisposes to drinking problems is no longer tenable but a number of personality traits which are manifest in childhood or in the teenage years are associated with a higher than average incidence of harmful drinking in adult life. They include hyperactivity, antisocial tendencies, impulsivity and extraversion. Sometimes the drinking problem is one of the manifestations of a definable personality disorder. Antisocial personality disorder occurs in 10 to 30 per cent of males with alcohol dependence and borderline personality disorder in 5 to 20 per cent of females. Diagnosis depends on a careful, historical assessment. It must be remembered that personality deterioration is often a sequel to alcohol dependence.

Psychiatric disorders

Several psychiatric disorders are associated with harmful drinking, but determining whether the relationship is a causal one is rendered difficult by the spectrum of mood disturbance and psychotic symptomatology that occurs in the withdrawal syndrome or is otherwise secondary to the drinking problem. A careful lifetime psychiatric history taken in conjunction with the drinking history will, in many cases, define whether a psychiatric disorder antedated the development of alcohol dependence, but where the picture is still clouded, reassessment after three to four weeks total abstinence from alcohol is essential. There is a marked sex-related difference in the frequency and nature of underlying psychiatric disorders; overall they are more common in women (occurring in 15 to 40 per cent), particularly generalised anxiety disorder, phobic disorder and minor and major depressive disorder. An underlying schizophrenia is more commonly seen in men, though the overall prevalence is only about twice that of the general population.

Life events

Although it would be simplistic to ascribe the development of a drinking problem to a specific event in a person's life, there are many instances where it seems to have started after a major trauma such as a bereavement. More often the effect is to facilitate a lifestyle involving heavy drinking. Examples include a new job in an outback community, working as a bartender, divorce with a consequent loosening of social ties and constraints.

Environmental factors

The overall availability of alcohol in a community, the social acceptability of heavy drinking and the constraints on this are potent factors in determining the prevalence of problem drinking in a particular community. The ready acceptance of heavy drinking and drunkenness by young men in country areas contributes to a high rate of problems among this cohort, though the distinction between country and city youth now seems to be less. The introduction of random breath testing has been followed by a gratifying reduction in fatal road accidents in many countries and the advent of low alcohol beers may have a similarly beneficial effect.

Examination

Mental state examination

Particular attention should be paid in the mental state examination to the following:

(a) clouding of consciousness;
(b) abnormalities of perception, especially visual and auditory hallucinations;
(c) abnormalities of thought, especially paranoid ideation;
(d) affect-anxiety, dysphoria, depression, blunting, lability;
(e) suicidal ideation;
(f) cognition, including awareness of current events, immediate recall, short-term and long-term memory; abstraction, conceptualisation and planning.

Formal cognitive function testing should await the resolution of any clouding of consciousness. The Short Mental Status Examination questionnaire is used by some as a simple screening instrument for alcohol-related brain damage. More sensitive screening procedures make use of a short battery of tests, usually under the direction of a clinical neuropsychologist.

Physical examination

Some physical indicators of harmful drinking have been presented in Table 7.3. A complete assessment should include the following:

(a) general appearance — evidence of premature ageing, Cushingoid facies;
(b) signs of intoxication—alcohol on breath, garrulousness, ataxia;
(c) cutaneous stigmata of harmful alcohol consumption such as facial telangiectasia, rhinophyma, thinning of skin, Dupuytren's contractures, bruises (especially of differing ages) and non-surgical scars;
(d) cutaneous stigmata of liver disease such as spider naevi, palmar erythema;
(e) signs of withdrawal—tremor and sweating of hands, tremor of face and tongue;
(f) pulse rate and blood pressure;

(g) evidence of cardiac enlargement/failure;
(h) size and consistency of liver, presence of splenic enlargement or of ascites;
(i) evidence of head injury;
(j) presence of nystagmus or ophthalmoplegia;
(k) ataxia, especially of stance and gait;
(l) signs of peripheral neuropathy.

Aids to diagnosis

Screening tests

Several screening tests are available to aid in the detection of alcoholism or harmful drinking, both among those attending hospitals or clinics and among the general population. They include the Michigan Alcoholism Screening Test (MAST), a 25-item questionnaire of which a number of abbreviated and self-administered versions now exist, the CAGE and the recently developed WHO screening instrument.[2] The MAST and the CAGE are described in Chapter 6. Both are efficient at detecting classical alcoholics but detect only 40 to 50 per cent of people with less severe problem drinking.

Screening procedures combining questionnaire items, clinical findings and/or laboratory tests (described in more detail below) have also been introduced recently. Examples are the Munich Alcoholism Test (MALT) and the Alcohol Clinical Index.[3] Both show considerable promise, though the former is a relatively complex procedure.

Laboratory investigations

Abnormalities of several biochemical and haematological parameters occur in persons with a hazardous alcohol consumption. Among these 'markers' are the erythrocyte mean cell volume ('MCV'), the serum aminotransferases (aspartate ['AST'] and alanine ['ALT']), serum gamma glutamyltransferase (gamma GT), uric acid, HDL-cholesterol and desialotransferrins. The likelihood of subjects with hazardous or harmful alcohol consumption having an abnormal test result increases with the age of the individual and with the chronicity and regularity of the drinking. Laboratory tests are more sensitive markers in patients attending medical units (40 to 90 per cent sensitivity) than those seen in psychiatric units, in private practice or in the population at large (10 to 50 per cent). A positive blood or breath alcohol reading is found in 10 to 40 per cent of persons with drinking problems. This finding can be used subsequently to confront the patient.

The sensitivity and specificity of the individual tests are not sufficiently high for any one to be used on its own as a screening procedure. Combinations of tests have been shown to distinguish persons with harmful alcohol consumption from normal drinkers with an accuracy exceeding 80 per cent, and are especially precise if weighted values based on discriminant functions are used.

In clinical practice the value of these tests is not so much in formal screening procedures but in raising the level of awareness that alcohol might be a problem and, in combination with items from the history and examination, in providing evidence of a person's harmful alcohol consumption. They are also useful in monitoring the response to intervention.

Assessment and diagnostic instruments

In specialist alcohol problems services, assessment and diagnostic instruments are widely used to supplement clinical information and to help the clinician formulate the most appropriate goals and interventions. 'Quantity-frequency-variability' interview schedules and questionnaires may be used to elicit quantitative information about alcohol intake. The severity of dependence on alcohol can be assessed by a self-administered questionnaire such as the Severity of Alcohol Dependence Questionnaire (SADQ)[4] referred to in Chapters 3 and 6. A comprehensive assessment instrument, termed 'A Structured Addictions Assessment Interview for Selecting Treatment' (ASIST) is produced by the Addiction Research Foundation, Toronto, Canada.

CHAPTER 8

Medical Aspects of Management: Therapy

John B. Saunders

In this chapter the medical approaches used in the management of the problem drinker are presented in chronological order, that is in the order that they may be required in the management of an individual patient. Firstly, the need for detoxification is considered and the drugs and treatments involved in this process are described. Following this there is an outline of treatment for complicating (or coexisting) psychiatric syndromes, for physical complications and of the underlying alcohol problem, particularly those techniques that fall within the province of the non-specialist physician.

Detoxification

Introduction

Persons who are physically dependent on alcohol are likely to go into withdrawal when they cease or reduce their consumption. Typically, the withdrawal syndrome starts 6 to 24 hours after the last drink. In some individuals the syndrome is short-lived and of little consequence. In others, particularly those with coexisting medical disorders, the withdrawal syndrome progresses to delirium tremens (DTs), an acute organic brain syndrome.

Detoxification is the process by which alcohol-dependent persons recover from the intoxicating effects of alcohol in a supervised way so that withdrawal symptoms and the risk of developing delirium tremens are minimised.

The setting for detoxification

It is often necessary for a person who seeks detoxification and/or is in withdrawal to be admitted to a clinic or hospital, but detoxification may be undertaken at home, provided that:

(a) there are no signs of severe withdrawal (severe tremor, fits, clouding of consciousness or hallucinations) at the time;

(b) there is no past history of delirium tremens or recurrent withdrawal fits;
(c) there are supportive relatives who could stay with the patient during the period of detoxification, supervise any medication and call for help when necessary;
(d) there are no medical illnesses such as pneumonia or pancreatitis or major coexisting diseases such as diabetes;
(e) there is no evidence of suicidal ideation; and
(f) the patient does not have access to alcohol.

Admission should be arranged for patients who have a history of severe withdrawal episodes, current signs of marked withdrawal, coexisting medical or psychiatric disorders or unfavourable domestic circumstances.

Monitoring withdrawal

Close supervision of patients in withdrawal is essential. Many in-patient facilities use a rating scale. One such is the 'Alcohol Withdrawal Symptoms Rating Scale' (AWS) developed at Royal Prince Alfred Hospital by W. Goodin (Fig. 8.1). In the AWS seven parameters are scored on a scale from 0 to 4. A score of up to 4 indicates a mild withdrawal syndrome, 5 to 9 moderate withdrawal, 10 to 14 severe withdrawal and 15 plus very severe withdrawal. Monitoring every four hours is advisable and if the score reaches 10, every two hours.

Indications for medication

The point at which sedatives should be prescribed depends both on the severity of withdrawal and also on the setting in which detoxification is taking place. In patients undergoing treatment in a purpose-built detoxification unit, it is my practice to withhold drugs until the score reaches 8 . However, patients in a highly distracting environment, such as a psychiatric admissions ward or an acute surgical ward, benefit from sedation once the withdrawal score is 5 or more. Patients in whom the AWS score is increasing rapidly should also be sedated. When detoxification is undertaken at home (where systematic monitoring is not possible), sedation may be initiated at the onset of withdrawal.

The dose of sedative should be titrated against the severity of the patient's withdrawal syndrome. *Drugs should not be given to patients who are still intoxicated.* The dose is highest in the first 48

FIGURE 8.1 Alcohol withdrawal scale

ITEM 1 PERSPIRATION 0 No abnormal sweating. 1 Moist skin. 2 Localised beads of sweat, e.g. on face, chest, etc. 3 Whole body wet from perspiration. 4 Profuse maximal sweating: clothes, linen, etc. are wet.	ITEM 2 TREMOR 0 No tremor. 1 Slight intentional tremor. 2 Constant slight tremor of upper extremities. 3 Constant marked tremor of extremities.
ITEM 3 ANXIETY 0 No apprehension or anxiety. 1 Slight apprehension. 2 Apprehension or understandable fear, e.g. of withdrawal symptoms. 3 Anxiety occasionally accentuated to state of panic. 4 Constant panic-like anxiety.	ITEM 4 AGITATION 0 Rest normally during day, no signs of agitation. 1 Slight restlessness, cannot sit or lie still, awake when others asleep. 2 Moves constantly, looks tense, wants to get out of bed but obeys requests to stay in bed. 3 Constantly restless, gets out of bed for no obvious reason, returns to bed if taken. 4 Maximally restless, aggressive, ignores request to stay in bed.
ITEM 5 AXILLA TEMPERATURE 0 Temperature of 37.0°C. or less. 1 Temperature of 37.1°- 37.5°C. 2 Temperature of 37.6°- 38.0°C. 3 Temperature of 38.1°- 38.5°C. 4 Temperature above 38.5°C.	ITEM 6 HALLUCINATIONS 0 No evidence of hallucinations 1 Distortions of real objects. Aware that these are not real if this is pointed out. 2 Appearance of totally new objects or perceptions, aware that these are not real if this is pointed out. 3 Believes the hallucinations real but still oriented in place and person. 4 Believes himself to be in a totally non existent environment, preoccupied and cannot be diverted or reassured.

ITEM 7 ORIENTATION

0 The patient is fully oriented in time, place and person.

1 The patient is oriented in person but is not sure where he is or what time it is.

2 Oriented in person but disorientated in time and place.

3 Doubtful personal orientation, disoriented in time and place; there may be short periods of lucidity.

4 Disoriented in time, place and person, no meaningful contact can be obtained.

Score

Up to 4:	Mild withdrawal syndrome
5 to 9 :	Moderate withdrawal syndrome
10 to 14 :	Severe withdrawal syndrome
15+ :	Very severe withdrawal syndrome

hours; after that it is reduced in a stepwise fashion and stopped after five to ten days. Only in exceptional circumstances should sedatives be continued after two weeks; there is a high risk of dependence. The drugs most commonly used for detoxification are chlormethiazole, and the benzodiazepines diazepam and chlordiazepoxide. The first two have the advantage of being anticonvulsants. The clinician is well advised to become familiar with just one of these drugs.

Drug therapy

Diazepam, a benzodiazepine tranquilliser, is the most commonly used sedative. It has a long half-life (of 18 to 40 hours) and the half-life of its biologically active metabolite desmethyldiazepam averages two to five days. Diazepam can therefore be given as a series of loading doses, following which it is usually unnecessary to prescribe any more. However, some clinicians prefer to give it on an interval basis. Suitable regimes are described in Table 8.1.

For patients in severe withdrawal an IV injection of 10 to 20 mg diazepam should be given over five minutes, followed, if necess-

TABLE 8.1
Sedative Regimes for Detoxification

Drug	Severity of withdrawal	Dosage and frequency	Comments
Chlormethiazole (Hemineurin)	Mild (AWS score 1-4)	If considered necessary, 1-2 capsules or tablets every 6 hours. Extra night time sedation may be needed.	Sedation not necessary in quiet surroundings, but may be indicated for patients in highly distracting environments, or who are immobilised or undergoing investigations.
	Moderate to severe (AWS score 5-14)	Commence with 2-4 capsules or tablets every 4-6 hours. An extra dose may be needed 2 hours after the first one. No more than 16 capsules or tablets should be given during the first 24 hours. Day 2: 2-3 capsules or tablets every 4-6 hours Days 3-4: 1-2 capsules or tablets every 4-6 hours Days 5-6: 1 capsule or tablet every 4-6 hours	Exact dosage and frequency will depend on severity of withdrawal, body weight and presence of coexisting physical disease (*vide infra*). Adjust dosage according to response. An alternative regime involving hourly administration of the drug is used in some centres and is described in 'Drug Treatment in Alcoholism'.[1]
	Very severe (AWS score 15+)	Intravenous infusion of 0.8% chlormethiazole edisylate. Give 25-100 ml over 5 minutes, then 2.5-5 ml/minute until sedation achieved. No more than 200 ml should be given over first 30 minutes. Maintenance dose: 0.5-1 ml/minute to maintain light sleep.	Exact dosage will depend on body weight and response. Danger of respiratory depression. Infusion must be administered using a drip monitor or infusion pump. Nurse patient in high dependency unit.

		SPECIAL SITUATIONS *The patient with chronic liver disease*	Take care that the patient has alcohol withdrawal and not hepatic encephalopathy. Consult specialist physician.
		(i) Cirrhosis: dose should be halved.	Bioavailability increased two- to four-fold because of impaired first-pass metabolism.
		(ii) Alcoholic hepatitis: Maintain usual unless (1) evidence of underlying cirrhosis or (2) severely deranged liver function (bilirubin>100μmol/1 or albumin <30g/1) when give half the usual dose.	Blood flow may be increased in alcoholic hepatitis – first pass metabolism normal or accelerated.
		The patient with chronic airflow limitation (i) without respiratory failure: dose should be halved. (ii) with respiratory failure: *do not sedate*.	Consult specialist physician. Ensure resuscitation facilities are available.
		The patient on no oral intake IV infusion may be used, at a rate of 1-5 ml/min., reducing to 0.5-1 ml/min. after sedation achieved. Alternatively give IM chlordiazepoxide *(vide infra)*.	An infusion rate within this range will usually be sufficient for moderate to severe withdrawal. For patients with delirium tremens, see above
The Benzodiazepines: Diazepam (Valium; Ducene)	Mild (AWS score 1-4)	If necessary (see above) 5-10 mg every 6-8 hours	
	Moderate to severe (AWS score 5-14)	*Alternative Regimes* (a) First 24 hours: 10-20 mg orally every 6 hours. An extra dose may be needed mid-way between the first two regular ones. Days 2-4: 10 mg every 6 hours. Days 5-6: 5 mg every 6 hours.	Dosage will depend on severity of withdrawal, body weight and presence of any physical disease.

Drug	Severity of withdrawal	Dosage and frequency	Comments
		(b) Loading dose(s): 20 mg every 2 hours until sedation achieved, then stop. Review after 4 hours. No more than 120 mg should be given in the first 12 hours.	An increasingly popular regime. Because of the long duration of action of diazepam, the dose given to produce initial sedation will usually suffice to cover the entire withdrawal syndrome.
		Subsequent days (usually unnecessary): 5-10 mg every 6 hours if needed.	
(Diazepam injection; Diazemuls)	Very severe (AWS score 15+)	Intravenous injection of 10–20 mg, repeated if necessary in the first 30 minutes. Maintenance dose of 1-5 mg/hour may be needed.	Danger of apnoea in first 2-3 minutes after administration. Beware of accumulation of drug. Nurse patient in high dependency unit.
		SPECIAL SITUATIONS *The patient with chronic liver disease* Cirrhosis or severe alcoholic hepatitis: dose should be halved.	Take care that the patient has alcohol withdrawal and not hepatic encephalopathy. Consult specialist physician. See guidelines for chlormethiazole.
		Alternatively use 15 mg oxazepam every 3 hours to a maximum of 45 mg, then review.	Beware of high abuse potential of oxazepam.
		The patient with chronic airflow limitation (i) without respiratory failure: dose should be halved. (ii) with respiratory failure: *do not sedate*.	Consult specialist physician. Ensure resuscitation facilities are available.

		The patient on no oral intake Give 10 mg IV followed by 1-5 mg/hour as necessary.	
Chlordiazepoxide (Librium)	Mild (AWS score 1-4)	If necessary (see above) 5-15 mg every 6 hours.	
	Moderate to severe (AWS score 5-14)	First 24 hours: 20-50 mg every 2-4 hours until withdrawal controlled. Then 20-50 mg every 6 hours. Days 2-4: 10-20 mg every 6 hours. Days 5-6: 5-10 mg every 6 hours.	Dosage and frequency will depend on severity of withdrawal, body weight and presence of any physical disease. Note that chlordiazepoxide has minimal anticonvulsant properties.
	Very severe (AWS scale 15+)	Intramuscular injection: 25-100 mg, repeated if necessary, in 2-4 hours.	This preparation is not available in Australia.
Major tranquillisers Haloperidol (Serenace)	Mild/ moderate	Not indicated.	They lower the seizure threshold, may cause hypotension and have no place in routine management.
	Severe withdrawal with hallucinations	By mouth: 2.5-5 mg, repeated once after 1 hour if necessary, then 1-5 mg every 6 hours thereafter, as indicated. Intramuscular or intravenous injection: 0.5-2 mg for mildly disturbed patient; 5-10 mg for severely disturbed one, repeated every hour for four hours if necessary, then 1-5 mg every 6-8 hours thereafter, as indicated.	Should be used as an adjunct to chlormethiazole or a benzodiazepine.

ary, by two further doses over the next half hour. A maintenance dose of 1 to 5 mg per hour (gradually reducing) by intravenous infusion may be necessary over the first 24 hours. Transient apnoeic episodes are well recognised after intravenous injection of benzodiazepines; the clinician should be present for at least 15 minutes after they are given. The patient should be in a high dependency unit.

Chlordiazepoxide is popular in the USA, but less so elsewhere. It has only weak anticonvulsant properties. The oral dosage ranges from 20 to 40 mg per day in mild cases of withdrawal to 200 to 800 mg per day for delirium tremens. It is usually given on an interval basis, six to eight hourly and after the first 48 hours may be tailed off fairly rapidly because of its relatively long half-life (averaging 20 hours). A parenteral preparation is available in the USA.

Chlormethiazole is a short acting sedative and anticonvulsant which is widely prescribed for alcohol withdrawal in the UK, Europe and Australasia but is not available in the USA. The oral preparation comes in the form of tablets or capsules, depending on the country. The dosage in the first 24 hours varies from 4 to 16 tablets or capsules; suitable regimes are outlined in Table 8.1. It is not advised for outpatient use because of its dependency potential. Chlormethiazole is also available in an intravenous preparation (of the edisylate salt) for patients with very severe withdrawal syndromes (for example, delirium tremens) or for those on no oral intake. Guidelines to its use are also given in Table 8.1. Intravenous chlormethiazole carries a significant risk of respiratory depression and reduction in the gag reflex; there have been several fatalities where patients have not been monitored adequately and all patients on intravenous chlormethiazole should be managed in high dependency units.

Barbiturates have no place in the management of alcohol withdrawal nowadays.

Major tranquillisers are no longer first line drugs for the management of alcohol withdrawal, having been superceded by the benzodiazepines. Adverse side effects include hypotension and a reduction in seizure threshold. Major tranquillisers should be reserved for patients with hallucinosis that has not responded to a conventional sedative regime. A suitable dose is 2.5 to 10 mg haloperidol ('Serenace') repeated at hourly intervals up to four times as necessary, then 1 to 5 mg every six hours.

Beta adrenergic blocking drugs are inferior to sedatives in the management of alcohol withdrawal. They may have a place as an adjunct to sedatives, but since there is at least a theoretical risk of induction of hypoglycaemia, there would seem little merit in adding them to a sedative regime.

Other aspects of management

The right environment

Persons in alcohol withdrawal are liable to overreact to what is happening in their immediate environment and become excessively agitated. Persons in incipient DTs readily incorporate external events into their confused, delusional or hallucinatory state. Relief of withdrawal symptoms is aided by the right setting and by appropriate counselling techniques. A few guidelines are provided:

1. The patient should be cared for in a quiet, non-stimulating, non-threatening and safe environment.
2. The therapist should employ a slow, steady, unthreatening approach to reduce anxiety, and avoid confrontation and arguments.
3. The counsellor should speak slowly and distinctly in a friendly manner.
4. When speaking there should be continuous eye to eye contact.
5. All interventions should be explained clearly.
6. Use touch to allay the patient's distress and anxiety.
7. Test the patient's reality base and orientation repeatedly and, if necessary, reacquaint the patient with his environment.
8. Try to explain the unreal nature of illusions and incipient hallucinations and try to distract the patient when delusions are causing anxiety.
9. A night light reduces the likelihood of perceptual errors and an exacerbation of anxiety and psychotic phenomena during the night.
10. When coercion is needed, clear direction should be given to the patient, but when he or she is endangering their life or threatening others physical restraint will be necessary. This should be employed with minimum force.

Vitamins

All patients in alcohol withdrawal (and indeed all alcohol-dependent patients) should receive thiamine as prophylaxis against Wernicke's encephalopathy. An intramuscular dose of 100 mg thiamine should be given each day for one week. If IM administration is not possible, 100 mg thiamine should be given orally three times a day. A large dose such as this is necessary because oral thiamine is poorly and erratically absorbed in alcoholic patients. Deficiencies of other B complex vitamins and of vitamin C are not uncommon and an oral multivitamin preparation should be taken for a few days.

Fluids and electrolytes

Severe withdrawal is often accompanied by fluid depletion or, on occasions, fluid overload. The fluid status of patients must be carefully assessed and when necessary intravenous saline or dextrose-saline should be administered. *Dextrose solutions should not be given until the patient has received at least one dose of thiamine 100 mg parenterally, as a glucose load in a patient with borderline thiamine status is likely to precipitate Wernicke's encephalopathy.* Hypokalaemia and hypomagnesaemia are frequent concomitants of severe withdrawal and should be treated with the appropriate supplements of potassium (80 to 240 mmol/day) or magnesium (40 to 100 mmol/day).

Anticonvulsants

These are frequently prescribed for the treatment or prophylaxis of fits in alcoholic patients, though in only a minority are they indicated or likely to be effective. Fits occur in about 5 per cent of patients undergoing withdrawal and typically occur 6 to 48 hours after the last drink. They are centrencephalic in type and present with sudden loss of consciousness and a tonico-clonic convulsion; there is no aura. In patients undergoing medicated detoxification there is rarely an indication for additional anticonvulsant therapy as chlormethiazole and most benzodiazepines (but *excluding* chlordiazepoxide) have anticonvulsant as well as sedating properties. It is the author's practice to restrict the use of anticonvulsants to those patients who have been taking these drugs on a regular basis prior to admission, for patients who have a history of withdrawal fits but who for some reason are not being sedated and, necessarily, for patients with epilepsy not related to withdrawal.

Standard regimes such as phenytoin 300 mg daily, carbamazepine 200 mg three times a day or 400 mg sodium valproate three times a day are usually satisfactory. After a withdrawal fit, some authorities recommend a loading dose of 250 mg phenytoin given intravenously over five minutes, followed by 250 mg 12 hours later. This is of unproven efficacy. The author prefers to institute or increase conventional sedation.

The differential diagnosis of alcohol withdrawal and other acute brain syndromes

Sedative withdrawal

The features of sedative withdrawal are very similar to those of alcohol withdrawal but tend to be delayed in onset and more protracted. Detoxification should be undertaken using diazepam which exhibits cross-tolerance with other sedatives, and has the advantage of a long half-life. Between 20 and 120 mg should be given daily in divided doses for two to five days after which it can be tailed off over a similar period.

Intoxication from alcohol and other drugs

This is often overlooked as a cause of confusion and bizarre behaviour. Supportive care as for drug overdoses is usually all that is necessary. Rarely, resuscitation, ventilation, dialysis and inotropic agents are required.

Acute Wernicke's encephalopathy

This is characterised by confusion and disorientation, usually nystagmus and other cerebellar signs and occasionally ophthalmoplegia. Delusions and hallucinations are less common. It is a diagnosis that must not be missed. Thiamine 100 mg intramuscularly should be given immediately on suspicion of the diagnosis and at daily intervals for a week.

Subdural haematoma

This presents with clouding of consciousness and sometimes headache and lateralising neurological signs. Where confusion is unexplained, even the absence of neurological abnormalities, CT scan is indicated. If a subdural haematoma is evident, an urgent neurosurgical referral should be made.

Metabolic encephalopathy

Other causes of a confusional state include hypoxia, hypercapnia, electrolyte disturbance, hepatic encephalopathy, anaemia and sepsis (especially pneumonia). Treatment is that of the underlying disorder. Sedation may be necessary as a temporary measure but is contraindicated in patients with chest disease or liver disease.

Acute alcoholic hallucinosis

This is characterised by predominantly auditory hallucinations (usually voices making derogatory statements) in the setting of clear consciousness. The syndrome occurs both during periods of very heavy drinking and in withdrawal and may persist for several weeks after cessation of alcohol consumption. Treatment with major tranquillisers is usually necessary to afford relief of symptoms at least in the acute stage. A suitable regime is haloperidol 2.5 to 10 mg every six hours or thioridazine ('Melleril') 50 mg every six hours.

Schizophrenia

The diagnosis of an underlying schizophrenia rests primarily on the persistence of psychotic symptomatology well beyond the time when withdrawal symptoms have abated, and is strengthened by a lack of response to minor tranquillisers and, when present, the perceptual abnormalities and thought disorder that are characteristic of schizophrenia. Treatment of the psychosis once the patient is detoxified is no different to usual.

Management of anxiety and depression

Anxiety disorders

Anxiety, agitation and panic reactions are integral components of the alcohol withdrawal syndrome and, correspondingly, withdrawal (either the overt clinical syndrome or the 'sub-clinical' withdrawal that occurs within a few hours of stopping drinking) is the commonest cause of an anxiety state in alcohol dependent persons. The symptoms are promptly relieved by further consumption of alcohol and thereby constitute a powerful stimulus to continue drinking. Anxiety and agitation increase in severity over the first 24 hours of withdrawal (if this is untreated) and, in the majority of cases, gradually abate as the withdrawal syndrome resolves. In a significant minority, though, symptoms continue for a variable time after the physical manifestations such as tremor and sweating have disappeared. Approximately 20 to 40 per cent of alcohol dependent persons have an antecedent history of anxiety disorder, usually 'free-floating' (i.e. generalised, chronic) anxiety or phobic disorder. It would be simplistic to regard the anxiety disorder as the cause, necessarily, of their alcohol problem, but symptoms of anxiety tend to persist after detoxification in this group. Women are affected more than men.

Formerly, minor tranquillisers were prescribed extensively for anxiety states both during detoxification and for those which persisted. With the increasing evidence for the abuse and dependency potential of these drugs, the indications for their use have become increasingly restricted. It is my practice to limit treatment to a maximum of ten days for detoxification or to two weeks on any one occasion for those with persisting symptoms. Non-pharmacological therapies are to be preferred in the latter case. They are described in Chapter 11.

Depression

Dysphoria is common in the 'hangover' phase after a drinking session in non-dependent drinkers. It is an integral feature of the early stages of the alcohol withdrawal syndrome, though this fact is not widely recognised. Mood becomes depressed within a few hours of stopping drinking and this may precede or overshadow the physical manifestations of withdrawal. With resolution of the withdrawal syndrome there is a lifting of the mood in the majority of patients but approximately 20 to 30 per cent have persistent depression. The classification of post-detoxification depressive states is unsatisfactory. Some patients have a reactive depression related to a specific event such as marital breakdown, bereavement or unemployment, or to a general downward social drift. In up to 5 per cent a major depressive illness becomes apparent after the masking effect of the person's alcohol dependence has been removed.

The diagnosis of a depressive illness that requires antidepressant medication cannot usually be made with confidence until two to four weeks have elapsed after cessation of drinking. Many symptoms of major depression such as diurnal variation in mood, a sense of worthlessness, recrimination, early morning wakening and gastrointestinal disturbance are common to alcohol dependence. The importance of reassessment after a period of abstinence is threefold. Firstly, it avoids unnecessary antidepressant medication for the majority of patients whose depression is related to alcohol dependence/withdrawal and is therefore self-limiting. Secondly, alcohol dependent persons with major depressive illness need careful monitoring. Thirdly, prescribing antidepressant drugs for alcohol dependent patients who continue to drink heavily is useless and can be dangerous. Whether antidepressant medication is indicated for patients with less severe depression post detoxification is an unresolved issue. There have been few randomised controlled trials of antidepressants in depressed alcohol dependent subjects. The samples have generally been inadequate and the definition of the depressive syndrome unsatisfactory.

Alcohol dependent persons with depression of any type are at high risk of suicide and an assessment of any suicidal ideation is essential. Pointers to suicidal intent are similar to those in non-alcohol affected persons and include profound depressive symptomatology, a feeling of hopelessness and concrete plans to carry out the act. Faced with an alcohol dependent patient who has dysphoria or frank depression, the clinician must first decide whether admission for detoxification is necessary or whether this could be attempted on a domiciliary basis. Urgent admission is required for those with suicidal intent. When an underlying major depressive illness becomes apparent or in other cases where depression is severe and persistent, antidepressant medication should be instituted.

Tricyclic or tetracyclic antidepressants are the drugs of choice for both these situations. The therapeutic dose may need to be 50 to 100 per cent higher than in non alcohol dependent individuals because of the effects of hepatic enzyme induction. Monitoring of plasma levels should be undertaken whenever possible. Some alcohol dependent patients find the sedating properties of certain tricyclic drugs unacceptable and a non-sedating drug such as nortriptylene is often preferred.

Lithium should be reserved at present for patients with an underlying bipolar disorder. Compliance with treatment is often a problem and careful monitoring of blood lithium levels is a prerequisite.

Monoamine oxidase inhibitors are best avoided. Many alcoholic drinks contain tyramine and can precipitate a dangerous hypertensive crisis in patients on these drugs.

Treatment of physical disorders

Alcoholic liver disease

Alcoholic liver disease is second only to road trauma as the commonest cause of morbidity and mortality amongst heavy drinkers. It exists in three main forms: fatty liver, alcoholic hepatitis and cirrhosis. Alcoholic fatty liver can develop after seven to ten days of hazardous drinking and persists as long as alcohol intake remains high. In most cases it is asymptomatic but it may cause pain in the right side of the abdomen, nausea and vomiting, dyspepsia and occasionally cholestatic jaundice. It requires no specific therapy other than abstinence from alcohol and a nutritious diet which includes an adequate amount of protein.

Alcoholic hepatitis typically presents with jaundice, fever and pain in the right side of the abdomen. In more severe cases hepatic decompensation may occur, with the development of progressive jaundice, ascites, coagulation disturbances and hepatic encephalopathy. The mortality rate in these cases is 20 to 40 per cent. On the other hand, in up to 50 per cent of cases overall the lesion is asymptomatic.

Alcoholic cirrhosis is the stage when liver injury is permanent. Typically, patients present with weight loss, abdominal pain, ascites or sometimes acute variceal haemorrhage or encephalopathy. Only 30 to 50 per cent of patients are still alive five years after diagnosis, and the outlook is significantly worse for those who continue drinking. Liver cancer is a well-recognised complication.

The mainstays of treatment for both alcoholic hepatitis and alcoholic cirrhosis are abstinence from alcohol and a nutritious diet. There is no therapy that reverses the histological lesions and essentially treatment is directed towards the complications of the disease. *Ascites* is managed by sodium restriction (20 to 40 mmol sodium per day) and an aldosterone antagonist diuretic such as spironolactone (initial dose 100 mg daily); a loop diuretic such as frusemide may be necessary in addition. *Acute variceal haemorrhage* is a medical emergency and the patient should be admitted urgently to a medical unit. Immediate treatment involves restoration of the blood volume, and reduction in portal pressure by using vasopressin and/or nitroglycerine. Oesophageal tamponade with a Sengstaken-Blakemore tube may be necessary to stem the haemorrhage. Definitive management is by endoscopic sclerotherapy of the varices or portal vein decompression. Beta adrenergic blocking drugs may have a role in the long-term management of portal hypertension. *Hepatic encephalopathy* is treated by protein restriction (40 g daily) and either by lactulose, a non-absorbable oligosaccharide or neomycin, a non-absorbable broad spectrum antibiotic. Both drugs inhibit the formation of toxic nitrogenous compounds and their absorption into the systemic circulation.

Alcoholic pancreatitis

Alcoholic pancreatitis may be acute or chronic. The acute disease varies in severity from a mild illness with dyspepsia-like pain to a devastating illness with excruciating upper abdominal pain, severe fluid depletion, hypotension and renal failure. Admission to an acute general hospital is necessary for the more severely ill patients. Chronic pancreatitis is characterised by deep-seated epigastric pain which is exacerbated by alcoholic binges. Pain relief is problematical as many patients become dependent on opiate analgesics. Alternative methods of pain relief such as coeliac plexus block or nerve stimulation should be explored. Pancreatectomy is sometimes necessary. When the pancreas is severely damaged, deficiency syndromes can arise. Exocrine gland insufficiency results in digestive disturbances, steatorrhoea and malnutrition. Its treatment consists of pancreatic enzyme supplements and antacids. Endocrine insufficiency causes diabetes and may necessitate treatment with oral hypoglycaemic agents or insulin.

Alcoholic cardiomyopathy

Alcoholic cardiomyopathy typically presents with biventricular heart failure and supraventricular arrythmias. Treatment consists of bed rest, diuretics (spironolactone and frusemide), sodium restriction and, for patients with atrial arrythmias, digitalis. It is my practice not to recommend anticoagulation for patients with alcoholic cardiomyopathy (such treatment is usual for patients with non alcoholic disease), unless the likelihood of total abstinence is very high, because of the risks of interaction between alcohol and the anticoagulant medication, and uncertain compliance with treatment. Patients with any form of heart disease should be advised not to drink excessively in view of the risk of alcohol induced arrythmias.

Systemic hypertension
Hypertension is a recently described complication of hazardous alcohol consumption and as many as 30 per cent of cases of so called 'essential hypertension' may be related to alcohol.[2] Patients should be advised to abstain from alcohol, whereupon blood pressure will return to normal in the majority. Treatment of hypertension in alcohol dependent patients who continue to drink is almost always ineffective. In this situation, complex therapy with multiple agents is necessary to achieve some reduction of blood pressure and even then it is rarely brought to within normal limits.

Hypertension occurring during detoxification is rarely a clinical problem; if blood pressure exceeds 200/120 Hg, methyldopa 250 mg to 500 mg three times daily can be added to the sedative regime.

Alcohol-related brain damage
Chronic brain damage comprises two basic syndromes, an amnestic syndrome, the most severe form of which is Korsakoff's psychosis, and the 'frontal lobe syndrome'. The amnestic syndrome is caused by thiamine deficiency, although alcohol toxicity or withdrawal may have a facilitatory role. Approximately 50 per cent of patients have a history of Wernicke's encephalopathy and a residual amnestic syndrome is more likely in patients who received delayed or inadequate treatment. The characteristic defect is a loss of short-term memory but with preservation of immediate recall. The loss of short-term memory ranges from mild to profound and confabulation is a feature of the more severe defects. The frontal lobe syndrome is manifested by defects in abstract thinking, conceptualisation and planning. Its aetiology is uncertain but there is an association with long-term heavy

sessional drinking. It also exists in varying degrees of severity. The amnestic syndrome and the frontal lobe syndrome commonly coexist.

There are no drugs that reverse established structural brain damage and the capacity for recovery of the more severe lesions is limited. Treatment consists of providing a supportive, structured environment, preferably one with which the patient is familiar. Experimental approaches have included the use of memory retraining and occupational rehabilitation in an inpatient programme. Many patients with brain damage graduate successfully from the inpatient setting to semi-independent life in a hostel and some, even those with moderately severe lesions, return to the community and maintain an abstinent lifestyle. On the other hand, severely damaged patients usually require nursing home or hostel accommodation, or even long-term placement in a psychiatric hospital.

Management of the underlying alcohol problem

Attention has been devoted so far to the management of complications of alcohol consumption. It is now appropriate to focus on the management of the underlying drinking problem.

Developing commitment

A crucial stage in the process of recovery is the development of commitment by the subject to modify his (or her) drinking behaviour. The physician has a major role to play at this stage by presenting the patient with objective evidence of alcohol related harm and emphasising the benefits of abstaining from alcohol or, in selected cases, in learning controlled drinking. The following points are among those the physician may bring up with the patient:

1. The calculated level of daily alcohol intake and the risks associated with that level of consumption.
2. The results of the physical examination; this might include the presence of cutaneous stigmata of excessive alcohol consumption, the finding of hepatomegaly, cardiomegaly, peripheral neuropathy, cerebellar disease and endocrine disturbance.
3. Evidence of alcohol related brain damage, from clinical cognitive function testing or neuropsychological assessment.

4. Results of laboratory tests which are markers of excessive alcohol consumption (these include the serum gamma glutamyl transferase activity, the serum transaminases and mean cell volume).
5. Results of the investigations of liver disease, cardiac disease or neuropathy, as appropriate.

A useful technique at this point is to draw a 'profit and loss account'. The patient should be asked to list the reasons why he would benefit from abstaining or controlling his drinking. Spontaneous responses might include a better relationship with the wife or girlfriend, having fewer arguments, fewer complaints at work or feeling healthier on waking each morning. The physician can then outline the benefits from modifying drinking behaviour including recovery from physical disease and relief of symptoms.

The setting of goals

Specific drinking goals should then be established. The physician should not seek to impose goals on an unwilling patient; the goals must be agreed on by clinician and patient alike and it is crucial for the patient to accept the responsibility of recovering from his alcohol problem. It is the physician's role to reinforce sensible decisions and steer the patient away from foolish ones that would commit him to an unworkable goal or one that is inappropriate for the degree of physical or psychological harm.

The issue of whether alcohol dependent persons can resume 'normal' or 'controlled' drinking has aroused considerable controversy. My own practice is to have the patient work towards a goal of total abstinence if he is physically dependent on alcohol or has major alcohol related disorders. Operationally, this translates into an abstinence goal for patients who:

(a) have suffered physical withdrawal symptoms at frequent intervals (weekly or more) for at least six months;
(b) have experienced severe withdrawal tremors, fits or delirium tremens at any stage;
(c) have chronic physical sequelae such as cirrhosis, pancreatitis or alcohol related brain damage;
(d) have coexisting major psychiatric illness;
(e) have antisocial or borderline personality disorder;

(f) have a highly impulsive and/or self-destructive pattern of drinking;
(g) have repeatedly failed at controlled drinking;
(h) have abstained for a period of at least six months in the past,
(i) or express the wish to abstain completely.

Alcohol sensitising drugs

Alcohol sensitising drugs are a valuable adjunct to treatment and are an integral component of many successful programmes. The prototype drug disulfiram ('Antabuse') was introduced over 30 years ago and since then short-acting analogues such as calcium carbimide ('Abstem') and long-acting ones such as nitrefazole have been developed. Their therapeutic effect is based on the expectation of an unpleasant flushing reaction after alcohol is taken. Alcohol sensitising drugs inhibit hepatic aldehyde dehydrogenase. If alcohol is taken, there is an accumulation of its principal metabolite, acetaldehyde, a noxious compound which triggers the flushing reaction. The flushing reaction affects the face and upper trunk and is accompanied by nausea and vomiting, palpitations and on occasions, hypotension and prostration. It usually occurs within 10 minutes of taking alcohol and reaches a peak at 20 to 30 minutes; it rarely lasts for more than one and a half hours. It varies in intensity between individuals and about 20 per cent do not have a clinically significant reaction on standard doses of the drug.

Disulfiram causes inhibition of enzyme activity within 12 hours and this is irreversible; recovery of enzyme activity depends on *de novo* synthesis. A reaction may occur up to five or six days after the drug was last taken. Calcium carbimide inhibits enzyme activity within an hour, the inhibition is reversible and lasts approximately 12 hours. The reaction is qualitatively similar to the disulfiram reaction but is less severe.

The theoretical rationale for alcohol sensitising drugs at the time of their introduction was that a conditioned aversive response to alcohol would develop after repeated flushing reactions. Some clinicians still attempt to induce an aversive reaction by giving small quantities of alcohol to the patient, but this is the exception nowadays. The basis for their therapeutic effect is, rather, the threat of an unpleasant reaction, which deters the subject from drinking. For a person who is facing the decision of whether to remain abstinent or restart drinking, the knowledge that an unpleasant reaction will occur after drinking alters the balance in favour of staying abstinent. The use of these drugs therefore facilitates the development of coping strategies for dealing with 'high risk' times. Disulfiram is particularly useful in this regard because its prolonged duration of action ensures that alcohol cannot be taken safely for several days after treatment has been discontinued.

Alcohol sensitising drugs are appropriate for patients who wish to abstain from alcohol and

(a) who feel the need for an external aid to maintain abstinence;
(b) who accept the idea of drug therapy to achieve this end; and
(c) in whom there are no medical or psycho-social contraindications.

Results of treatment are better in those who have friends or relatives to provide support for abstinence, particularly if such a person can supervise the drug being taken as part of a contractual agreement.

Before treatment is commenced the patient must be fully informed of the objectives, the mechanism of action of the drug and the nature of the reaction. If the patient has not taken a drink for twenty-four hours, the initial dose may be given at the time of consultation. This is a useful test of the patient's motivation to abstain and commitment to take the drug. The starting dose of disulfiram is 500 mg daily (for one week) followed by 250 mg daily thereafter. The usual dose of calcium carbimide is 50 mg twice daily. Alcohol sensitising drugs are not a cure for alcohol problems in themselves and should be part of an overall therapeutic strategy which might include attendance at Alcoholics Anonymous, or placement in an abstinent environment. A typical length of treatment is three to six months, during which time the patient should aim to develop the personal resources to maintain abstinence in the long term after the drug has been stopped.

Contraindications to the use of alcohol sensitising drugs include a history of cardiac arrythmias, heart disease, uncontrolled hypertension, cirrhosis with portal hypertension, advanced pulmonary disease, pregnancy, schizophrenia, severe depression or treatment with alpha- or beta-adrenergic blockers, vasodilators, tricyclic antidepressants, monoamine oxidase inhibitors or phenothiazines. They are also best avoided in patients who have a very impulsive and explosive pattern of drinking, though each case must be judged on its individual merits.

Working with other services

Once a person has been identified as having a drinking problem and the initial therapy has been undertaken (together with any necessary detoxification and medical treatment), a decision must be made as to the need for ongoing treatment and who will undertake this. There is a variety of public, private and non-governmental services and it is axiomatic that the clinician should have an adequate knowledge of such resources and be able to liaise with them. They include:

Drug and alcohol units in public hospitals

These are of three main types:

Services in psychiatric hospitals

These units typically provide an inpatient programme lasting several weeks and are based on psychotherapeutic principles. Many are being phased out at the present time or are being converted to manage patients with coexisting psychiatric disorders or alcohol related brain damage.

Specialist alcoholism clinics

These hospitals cater solely for patients with alcohol (and sometimes drug) problems and usually provide both inpatient facilities (for detoxification and/or short-term rehabilitation programmes) and outpatient services.

Services in general hospitals

A development that has taken place over the last decade has been the establishment of alcohol and drug services in general hospitals. The emphasis is on outpatient treatment programmes, consultation-liaison services within the hospital and access to detoxification facilities and medical and psychiatric care where necessary. This trend is likely to continue.

Community public sector facilities

These are developed to a variable extent. In some areas there is a network of drug and alcohol workers based in community health centres, specialist drug and alcohol clinics or community detoxification centres. They provide the major public sector services. In other areas they are poorly developed.

Each type of service listed should optimally provide a multidisciplinary team consisting of psychiatrists, psychologists, counsellors, medical specialists and social workers. Comprehensive assessment and matching of the treatment strategy to the patient's needs should be available, through taking advantage of the multidisciplinary skills of the team.

Non-governmental agencies

Many non-governmental agencies provide a range of assessment and counselling facilities and some offer accommodation, structured rehabilitation programmes, education and vocational training, and legal advice. The clinician is well advised to have an index of these agencies and to make contact with some to facilitate the process of referral. Among the best known ones are the Salvation Army and Odyssey House. Some agencies provide services specifically for women or for ethnic minorities. A list of meetings of Alcoholics Anonymous, AlAnon and Alateen groups is available from the corresponding Central Service Office in major cities.

Current issues in management

The place of inpatient treatment programmes

The place of inpatient treatment programmes has been the subject of considerable, sometimes acrimonious, debate over the past 15 years. At one time these programmes, which were typically of two to three months' duration, were considered the optimal mode of treatment for patients with alcohol problems, especially those who had an established dependence. Their effectiveness has been called into question because of the high relapse rate of patients after discharge, and particularly since the influential studies of Edwards and colleagues[3,4] which demonstrated that inpatient treatment conferred no long-term benefits over a relatively simple outpatient approach.

Early intervention

The shift in emphasis away from prolonged inpatient programmes for patients with severe dependence is one result of a critical analysis of many traditional ways of treating persons with harmful alcohol consumption. Concentrating treatment efforts on severely damaged patients is not regarded as the most appropriate use of relatively limited resources. Specifically, the difficulty in inducing behavioural change in patients who have experienced major social decline or cognitive impairment, and the relatively poor prognosis for such patients has focussed on the need for intervention at an earlier stage. At this stage controlled drinking may be a viable option.

Results of trials of early intervention show considerable promise. Kristenson and Hood[5] identified problem drinkers amongst a cohort of middle-aged men through a combination of serum gamma GT and a questionnaire administered during a health screening programme. Subjects were randomised into an intervention group who received counselling and feedback of their laboratory results and a control group who were advised of their results but did not receive any systematic intervention. In the five years following admission to the study the rate of hospitalisation was reduced by 61 per cent in the group who received counselling; their mortality rate was halved. Chick and colleagues[6] in a study of patients admitted to medical wards in Edinburgh, Scotland, identified those with alcohol problems using a questionnaire. After randomisation half received advice to abstain from alcohol and problem solving strategies in a session lasting approximately 30 minutes, while the others received no advice. One year later those who had counselling had significantly less experience of alcohol problems and a greater reduction in serum gamma GT. This approach has been endorsed by WHO and a multicentre study of various types of early intervention is in progress.

New horizons in pharmacological therapies

There has been a resurgence of interest in pharmacological therapies for problem drinking, following a series of neurochemical studies in experimental animals which have demonstrated deficiencies in serotoninergic (and to a lesser extent dopaminergic) transmission following exposure to alcohol. Reduction in serotonin levels in the nucleus accumbens is found in rats selectively bred for their high spontaneous alcohol consumption. Clinical trials of the serotonin uptake inhibitors zimelidine and citalopram in problem drinkers have demonstrated reductions in the overall amount of alcohol consumed and especially in the number of drinking days.[7] Zimeldine has been withdrawn from the market because of side effects but clinical trials of citalopram and its analogues are continuing.

CHAPTER 9

Aversion Therapy

There are only a few books available about aversion therapy and nothing had been written for 20 years prior to Hadley's 1985 theoretical treatise. The reasons for the lack of contributions stated by Rachman and Teasdale, the authors of the latest clinical book on the subject,[1] still apply today. 'Most people have mixed feelings about aversion therapy. On the one hand we are interested in it as a psychological process and welcome the introduction of effective treatment procedures. On the other hand, we recognise it aş an unpleasant form of therapy and one which is open to abuse.'[2] Hadley expresses the same cautions in his book: 'Aversion therapy remains a sensitive issue on numerous accounts and it behoves the behavioural clinician (and all others) to proceed with caution'.[3] In the following pages we have tried to keep these reservations in mind. In the days of a more simple behaviourism, aversion therapy was used as though it was, by itself, a cure for alcoholism. The uncritical use of aversion therapy in the 1960s caused a reaction in the opposite direction. By the 1980s something like a balanced view has come to replace the earlier extremes of uncritical acceptance and blanket rejection. More importantly, the empirical studies and conceptual advances of recent years provide the basis for the incorporation of aversion therapy into a broad-spectrum treatment programme but there is little to which the practicing clinician can turn for conceptual and technical guidance in aversion therapy. Accordingly the following pages are designed to acquaint practitioners with new developments, novel applications of old procedures and the limitations as well as the potential applications of aversion therapy for problem drinking. Finally, new developments in behavioural biology and experimental psychology will be discussed and new treatment approaches based on these developments will be proposed.

The aims, procedures and concepts of aversion therapy for alcoholism can be stated simply: to reduce or eliminate drinking by aversive classical conditioning, which provides the patient with a painful or unpleasant stimulus immediately after making contact with the alcoholic drink. The stimulus presented first (whisky, beer, etc.) is termed the conditioned stimulus (CS) and the second, aversive, event is termed the unconditioned stimulus (UCS, which is usually an electric shock or an emetic drug). The theory states that after repeated pairings of the CS and the UCS within seconds of each other, and in that order, the innate response to the latter stimulus (anxiety to painful shock; nausea to emetic drugs) will be elicited by the former. In the typical arrangement, the patient is given alcohol to look at, smell and/or taste and then, immediately afterwards, a harmless but painful (non-convulsive) electric shock is delivered to the fingers or hand of the patient.

A second procedure, aversive operant conditioning, follows essentially the same steps except that there is usually some provision for the patient to spit out or to refuse the alcohol, at which point the therapist withholds or turns off the shock on that trial. There are, however, important theoretical differences between procedures in terms of the supposed mechanisms of change. In classical conditioning the goal is to produce a change in the incentive value of the alcohol CS; the drink should become less attractive. In aversive operant conditioning the goal is the elimination of the behaviour which is maladaptive (here, drinking).

Whichever procedure is adopted, the practicing therapist is faced with deciding which aversive stimulus to use. To date, this matter has received little systematic theoretical or empirical analysis. With few exceptions[4] those who discuss the problem at all offer commonsense criteria as a guide to clinical practice: first, aversive stimuli should pose no threat to the physical or psychological well-being of the patient and, second, aversive stimuli should, of course, be unpleasant to experience.

The most widely used aversive stimuli have been electric shock and emetic drugs, and so for most therapists the clinical decision about the administration of aversion therapy reduces to choice between these two classes of stimuli. In their influential book Rachman and Teasdale[5] strongly advocate the use of electric shock. As they see it, there are a number of serious disadvantages with the use of emetic drugs. Some patients are unable to tolerate them and in some few cases, with 'end stage' drinkers, they may prove to be lethal. Clinical staff typically find them unpleasant to administer and reactions to the drugs themselves can be unpredictable in the time of onset and the intensity of the response they produce. The advantages of electric shock are that it provides for greater safety and flexibility, and precise control over the onset, duration, offset and intensity of the aversive stimulus. Behaviour therapists attach great importance to procedures which give control over the onset of the reaction to the aversive UCS (the unconditioned response or the UCR).[6] This last point has received considerable emphasis because it is taken as an established fact that for conditioning to occur all CSs (alcohol or any other) must be followed within a second or two by the UCS (or, to be more exact, the UCR). Temporal contiguity is easy to arrange with electric shock but is almost impossible with drug aversive stimuli.

From the argument thus far it would seem that the case is established for electric shock as the ideal aversive stimulus, and one might imagine that the preference for shock rests on a mass of convincing data from clinical reports. Surprisingly, there is no clinical evidence to support either the belief in the superiority of electrical over chemical methods—if anything, the opposite is true—or the importance of precise temporal control (indeed there are no well controlled studies addressed to these questions, and very few of any kind, in the clinical literature). The choice of electric shock reflects the strong influence of traditional conditioning theory on the concepts and methods of aversion therapy. According to this theory, any stimulus will be transformed into a conditioned stimulus (CS) if it occurs a second or two before the onset of the unconditioned stimulus (provided a sufficient number of these pairings are carried out). Studies undertaken with animals and humans to test this proposition have invariably employed auditory or visual events as conditioned stimuli and electric shock as the aversive unconditioned stimulus. Though audiovisual stimuli are used for reasons of convenience it is assumed that what has been demonstrated for, say, lights or buzzers (as CSs) and shock (as the UCS) holds equally for all conditioned and unconditioned stimuli.[7] Conditioning theorists from Pavlov onwards have assumed this without question but, it should be stressed, it had not, until the 1970s, been systematically and rigorously investigated.

Behaviour therapists took their views from the conditioning laboratory directly into the clinic, hence their advocacy of electric shock. As they put it, what difference does the choice of aversive stimulus make, as long as there is a safe and noxious UCS which can be presented immediately following contact with the CS (alcohol)?

Two lines of evidence, one from recent animal studies and the other from older clinical work, suggest that the answer may very well be: it matters a great deal. To take the animal evidence first, Garcia and his co-workers have conducted a large number of experiments which show that the equal associability premise adopted by most behaviour therapists is incorrect. Consider a typical experiment from Garcia's laboratory. A thirsty animal is allowed to drink a palatable solution such as saccharin-flavoured water which it prefers to tap water. The animal is then injected with a nausea-producing drug (for example, lithium chloride). When it recovers from the illness, is again made thirsty, and is given access to the saccharin water, the animal consumes much less than it did on the first trial prior to illness. If there are a number of such pairings, saccharin will be refused wherever it is encountered. Furthermore, the interval between saccharin consumption and the sickness can be minutes or hours and conditioning will still occur.[8]

Contrast these findings with those from animal subjects who have had lights or tones instead of tastes paired with an illness-inducing drug. On recovery the animals show little, if any, avoidance to those lights or tones. However, those same cues make ideal conditioned stimuli when they precede and are paired with painful electric shock. When visual or auditory cues are paired with shock the effective CS-UCS interval is a very brief one, ideally less than a minute, and not the minutes or hours shown to be effective in taste-aversion studies. Lastly, rats and other animals do not learn aversions to foods or fluids when an electric shock is used as the aversive stimulus. While it is easy to suppress consumption of a food or fluid in a particular environment by presenting a shock whenever the animal eats or drinks there, what the animal appears to learn is an avoidance of the place where the aversive stimulus is presented instead of developing an aversion to the consumed substance itself. That is, the avoidance is situation-specific. The very same food or fluid presented in a different situation is readily accepted.[9]

To summarise these results, animals quickly learn to associate tastes with illnesses that follow the taste. Taste and shocks, or lights/tones and illness associations are learned with difficulty, if they can be acquired at all. (Birds may be exceptions here; at least some avian species can learn illness-based aversions to either tastes or colours.)[10]

Garcia has offered an evolutionary-biological framework within which to interpret these results. He argues that an adaptive advantage would be conferred on animals predisposed to link up the taste of a food or fluid, and not the sights and sounds incidental to consumption, with nausea and gastrointestinal disturbances. Furthermore since in the natural environment the consequences of ingestion can take minutes or even hours to develop, long delay learning is to be expected within this system. Contrast this with the expectation which this perspective provides when aversive stimuli are used which cause pain to the surface of the body. In the natural (as opposed to the lab) environment, a second or two after the sight or sound of a predator a painful assault may occur. It is unlikely that a predator would himself survive if he were to get close enough to be seen or heard and then wait minutes or hours to attack. Thus rapid but short delay conditioning should characterise this system. And since, in the usual course of events, exteroceptive (for example, lights, noises) stimuli are likely to be the best predictors of imminent danger, tastes (but not smells) should be poor candidates as conditioned stimuli in such situations. The experimental results reviewed earlier are perfectly consistent with these deductions from Garcia's theory.

To sum up, current research into the mechanisms of animal behaviour points to the existence of biological-structural constraints on learning that can be understood by considering not just the number and timing of CS-UCS pairings but also the way in which the animal functions in his evolutionary niche. The assumption of extreme associative plasticity advanced by traditional conditioning theories has not been upheld. Specifically, with regard to aversive conditioning, this work suggests that the UCS in some way works backward to 'select' the CSs with which it will associate. Illness UCSs associate preferentially with taste stimuli, whereas pain producing UCSs such as electric shock make auditory and visual events the most likely candidates for conditioning.

These findings call into question the maxims of aversion therapy based upon a view of conditioning which is now seriously in doubt. However, the work just reviewed has been confined to animals and thus cannot stand by itself as an indictment of the practice of traditional aversion therapy for alcoholism. As for the clinical literature, a clear picture is not available because very few well controlled studies have been carried out in the area. Nevertheless, such evidence as there is fits nicely with the taste-aversion literature and is consistent with the evolutionary-biological view of conditioning outlined above.

Therapists who have used chemical aversion methods to create nausea have achieved markedly higher success rates than have those who have attempted to condition aversions to alcohol by pairing it with electric shocks. By far the largest and most carefully conducted study to date was reported by Le Mere and Voegtlin,[11] ironically not long before aversion therapy went out of fashion. Over a 13-year period they treated more than 4000 fee-paying alcoholic inpatients at the Shadel Sanitorium in Seattle with 'conditioned reflex therapy'. Patients were given alcohol to look at, smell and taste, after which they were made ill by an injection of emetine, a drug which causes nausea and vomiting. Up to three such trials were held per session. All told there were about 12 trials carried out over the ten-day hospitalisation period. At the end of a one-year follow-up 60 per cent of the patients were abstinent. For those who received additional booster sessions, the abstinence figure climbed to 90 per cent. These results are very impressive but before accepting the conclusion that alcohol-nausea aversion therapy is a sure-fire cure it should be noted that other forms of help were given and, furthermore, that in the main their patients were middle-class fee-paying patients with a good prognosis. It is not possible, therefore, to know what part of this improvement to assign to the chemical aversive method used by Le Mere and Voegtlin.

In a more recent study Miller, Dvorak and Turner[12] adapted this method to a group context. They treated ten alcoholics in a group setting and at an eight-month follow-up only two of their patients showed a relapse. Miller et al. felt that seeing the others ill and vomiting after drinking added to the impact of the treatment. More recently, in a USSR study, Zvonikiev[13] did a clinical experiment along the same lines as Miller and his associates. Zvonikiev reported excellent results from 1100 chronic alcoholics who were treated in groups of 40 to 45. There are other reports which also point to the superiority of chemical over electrical aversion therapy for alcoholism.[14]

One notable and widely cited exception was reported by Wallerstein.[15] He found that alcohol-illness pairings were only moderately effective and no better than routine care. Before his results can be taken at face value it is important to note a serious flaw in Wallerstein's technique, in that he had nausea occurring *before* the taste. Once they were nauseous the patients were then given the alcohol to taste. Wallerstein hoped thereby to create an aversion to alcohol by causing an association to occur between it and emesis. Judging by the experimental literature on taste aversion learning, this was almost certainly a questionable strategy. On the evidence to date, the crucial event for the production of a conditioned taste aversion is nausea and not vomiting (rats, for example, can form robust conditioned taste aversions even though they are unable to vomit). Wallerstein's procedure, then, was a 'backward conditioning' arrangement, where the reaction caused by the UCS came before the CS. This is known to be ineffective, regardless of whether shocks, drugs or other UCSs are employed.[16]

A study just concluded in our laboratory raises even more serious questions about Wallerstein's procedure and others like it. Having nausea precede the taste may cause a 'medicinal' effect. This is a term coined by Garcia to describe the opposite reaction to a taste aversion. His theory says that a taste preceding nausea loses its incentive properties while one that follows nausea, and which is associated with its decline, gains incentive value. Our findings were exactly in line with Garcia's theory. Subjects were made ill, in this case by rapid rotation in a specially-designed chair, and then given a fluid to drink. Another different fluid was given prior to rotation-induced nausea. On another day they were tested when they had completely recovered from the nausea. The flavour that preceded nausea was rated significantly lower; the one given after nausea had reached its peak gained significantly in preference ratings. Therefore there is a real possibility that the best that Wallerstein could have accomplished with his patients was 'no change'; at worst he may have inadvertently enhanced the preference of the target drink by having his patients drink it following nausea.

Wallerstein's study apart, positive clinical outcomes from studies utilising electric shock are fewer than those employing nausea. In one of the best of these studies Blake[17] gave his patients shock after they tasted alcohol. The shock was turned off when the alcohol was spat out. This was done in an attempt to condition 'relief' to the rejection of alcohol. A one-year follow-up showed 23 per cent to be abstinent. For those patients who received relaxation therapy in addition, 46 per cent were abstinent. The added benefits of relaxation, which are discussed in detail in Chapter 11, point to the value of a 'broad spectrum' approach to the treatment of alcoholism where different therapies (aversion therapy, relaxation, counselling, etc.) are combined with and not pitted against each other. As for the 23 per cent success rate from those who received electrical aversion therapy, later reports[18] suggest that this may have been due more to patient attitudes and expectations than to the hoped-for conditioning of anxiety to alcohol.

Vogler, Lunde, Johnson and Martin[19] used an interesting measure of the effectiveness of their aversive (shock) classical conditioning treatment, which was the time taken to relapse following therapy. Some of their alcoholics received shock in a random relation to the consumption of alcohol and others received the conventional alcohol-shock pairings. The former method was given the name 'pseudo-conditioning' because the aversive shock was not paired with the alcohol. The theory underlying aversion therapy requires that, all other things equal, the conditioning (i.e. pairing) patients improve more than the pseudo-conditioning patients. The data show that on the key measure employed, rehospitalisation, these two groups did not differ.

In another well-controlled study, Marlatt[20] compared the outcomes in chronic hospitalised alcoholics of two groups treated with aversive shock (conditioning and pseudo-conditioning) with a no-treatment control group. At a 15-month follow-up there were no differences between these groups. These results, and others like them,[21] challenge the assumption that pairing alcohol with an aversive electric shock creates an aversion to the alcohol or, even, that however it works, it is an effective form of therapy.

This review has been illustrative rather than exhaustive (see Appendix B for a fuller discussion) but the consistency of the results across clinical and experimental areas supports the following conclusions. First, chemical, or more specifically, nausea aversion methods have, on the whole, proved to be more effective than aversive shock in changing the attractiveness of alcohol and its expected effects in problem drinkers. This, of course, is not the same as a 'sure cure' and we are convinced by the mass of good clinical research of the need for broad-spectrum approaches. Second, the selection of the correct aversive stimulus is a matter of fundamental importance.

It now seems apparent that a blanket recommendation for aversion therapy, regardless of the aversive stimulus, has to give way to analyses based on the relevance of the particular aversive stimulus to the problem. Shock, then, is no more to be rejected outright than it is to be given the status of 'the' aversive stimulus. (in the treatment of certain sexual deviations such as fetishism it has led to good results[22]). It is no more valid, either, to elevate chemical aversion procedures to the status once held by electric shock. The question so often posed in contemporary clinical debates—'chemical or electrical aversion?'—is not well stated because it puts the focus on the class of aversive stimulus instead of the effects it must produce (nausea). For example, Sanderson and his co-workers[23] paired alcoholic drinks with a curare-like drug which caused temporary and complete paralysis in their patients. This UCS was chemical and, without question, highly aversive. ('Terrifying' said the patients who thought they were victims of a faulty procedure which was going to cost them their lives.) Campbell and his co-workers were sharply censured for failing to tell their patients that they would be temporarily paralysed and unable to speak or breathe (they were told that it might be somewhat unpleasant). The results from the alcoholics who underwent these alcohol-drug sessions are even less impressive than those typically reported in shock aversion studies. The problem is that this method was not relevant to the aim, which was to produce a conditioned distaste—better, a visceral dislike—of alcohol. The question to ask is not 'should we use a chemical, or shock (or whatever) aversive UCS?' but rather 'what techniques are there which reliably induce a state of nausea or illness following the taste of alcohol (or food, in the case of obesity)?'

While the evidence reviewed here may appear to settle the question in principle, very serious practical problems can arise in the application of these ideas. Clinical accounts and animal studies indicate that it is more difficult to condition aversions to familiar than to novel substances, and clearly alcohol is familiar to alcoholics. This problem can be overcome by arranging for a sufficient number of alcohol (or food) illness sessions. But for patients in ill health even a few trials with strong emetic drugs may be too many.

A resolution of this dilemma may be possible by adherence to the principle that only procedures which cause gastrointestinal illness or nausea are candidates for use in aversion therapy treatments if the aim is to develop a conditioned aversion to some food or fluid. With animals, emetic drugs, x-rays and rotation have all been tested successfully to produce taste aversions. The first of these has been the only one of the three used by behaviour therapists and, as already noted, it brings along with it potential risks to the patient's health. The second is even more obviously not appropriate, but the third, rotation, and a fourth, covert sensitisation, merit consideration. (Disulfiram, 'Antabuse', causes extremely unpleasant reactions when paired with alcohol but nausea is not always among these.)

If animals are briefly and rapidly rotated around their own axis after eating or drinking, they will subsequently avoid the substance paired with that rotation.[24] Taste aversions produced in this fashion resemble those brought about by nausea generated through the use of potentially dangerous methods like x-ray irradiation and powerful emetic drugs. Exactly how this is accomplished in physiological or biochemical terms is still unclear. It is possible that despite their differences in modes of operation they operate via a final common path of gastrointestinal malaise. This is impossible to verify from animal experiments but people exposed to high levels of radiation, injected with emetic drugs or rapidly rotated, all describe the experience as nauseating. In any event, the mechanisms by which rotation causes taste aversions is of less importance to clinicians than the fact that the procedure is simple and safe, however often it is used.

As an example of how it functions, we will describe a typical case. The patient was a man of 46 who had been a heavy drinker for more than ten years. His goal was to stop drinking, at least for a year. He was a heavy beer drinker and occasionally he drank spirits or wine to intoxication. Beer was selected as the target stimulus. The patient was asked to look at, smell and taste his favourite beer for one minute. Then the specially designed chair in which he was seated was rotated for five minutes at a speed of about 80 revolutions per minute. Ten such pairings were carried out over two sessions. At the end of the second session he reported a strong revulsion to the taste and smell (but not the sight) of beer. At a six-month follow-up he said that he had been abstinent for the whole period with the exception of a few occasions of light drinking (not beer). This report was corroborated by his wife.

We will consider a collection of problems with and objections to aversion therapy but before that we must acknowledge the limitations of aversion therapy as a treatment modality for patients whose motivation to recover is weaker than their desire to continue drinking. Any person who wished to 'break through' such a strong aversion could do so by deliberately drinking the target alcoholic beverage to bring about extinction of the conditioned response. Clients who are reasonably intelligent, highly motivated and especially cooperative are all good candidates when abstinence is the outcome selected. In the case study outlined above, other forms of therapy (counselling, assertiveness training and relaxation) were also used, so the most sensible evaluation of the rotation procedure (or, for that matter, any other kind of aversion therapy) is that it appears to be a very useful adjunct to other approaches, if used correctly.

We have carried out extensive tests with a number of volunteer subjects. In these, rotation produced nausea in 95 cases out of 100, and did so within ten minutes. Two predictors of the efficacy of rotation as a UCS emerged from these tests. First, those who fail to experience nausea after ten minutes of continuous rotation will not do so at any time and are poor prospects for taste-aversion conditioning by this method. Second, and in line with the experimental work on animals, nausea, and not vomiting, is the response which must occur to the rotation if conditioning is to occur. Thus far, this procedure has promise where the clinical goal is to produce a conditioned aversion to alcohol. (The work with food is at a preliminary stage, but the results here are less encouraging. Problem drinkers, save perhaps for the 5 per cent which form the 'Skid Row' group, drink within a relatively narrow range, whereas if an obese person is averted to, say, chips, any one of hundreds of other foods can be substituted.)

Finally, it is strongly emphasised that the theoretical, technical and clinical issues raised here are not offered as answers to the difficult questions of judgement and ethics which inevitably confront the clinical practitioner in this area. But where it is decided to employ aversion therapy procedures in the treatment of alcoholism (and perhaps obesity too) the developments in behavioural biology and experimental psychology reviewed here offer new and important perspectives as a guide to the development and refinement of effective aversive procedures.

Objections, problems and precautions

Whenever we give the rationale and the results favouring the (judicious) use of aversion therapy a number of objections and questions are invariably encountered. We have found that the only way to promote cooperation among patients and overcome objections in fellow professionals is to take the time to deal carefully with misconceptions. The most common are discussed below.

Confusions over 'aversion' therapy

In their training, clinicians are made aware of the first and time-honoured principle of help giving: do no harm. Aversion therapy seems to strike at the heart of this principle. The belief that it is aversive and thus does do harm is rooted in the assumption that there are two general categories of therapy, 'aversive' and 'benign'. A further and obvious assumption is that benign techniques are to be preferred.

A closer examination of the aversive/benign dichotomy reveals that it cannot be sustained. As an example, take one of the 'benign-gentle' techniques, systematic desensitisation. It contains a number of components but the basic idea behind the therapy is to have individuals with phobic avoidance gradually confront the things which they avoid. In no system of classifying techniques is systematic desentisation listed as aversive. Patients will hold a different view. Dr Wayne Wardman, co-author of a book on agoraphobia, a condition he had had for ten years, remarked on hearing the outlines of exposure therapy via systematic desentisation: 'I felt caught between an intolerable treatment and an unendurable problem'.[25] Though not aversive to the clinician, it certainly was to him, despite the reductions in phobic anxiety. As another example, pressing patients to recall traumatising material may be necessary but the process of bringing it to the surface can cause deep anguish. Counselling parents to withhold a desired but harmful substance from a child may well be aversive for the youngster but necessary for his emotion wellbeing. More examples could be given but the point is made. Aversive is a word that describes the patient's reactions to events and is not a label for a collection of techniques. Use of the more specific words 'painful' or 'nauseating' can help to avoid the false dichotomy.

Regarding aversion therapies as a homogeneous group
Attempts have been made to evaluate 'the' efficacy of aversion therapy. The obstacle to drawing general conclusions about aversion therapy is that 'aversive' techniques which have an established record of value in one area of therapy may be of no value at all in others. Electric shock techniques have been used with great success in eliminating self-injurious behaviour in deeply disturbed autistic children. Unless straitjacketed, either physically or through the use of drugs, these hospitalised children would smash their heads into hard surfaces, attempt to bite off their fingers or tear at their own skin. (Such children are unable to make use of language in any way, so psychotherapy is out of the question.) Two researchers, a psychologist and a psychiatrist at the University of California decided to use an aversive conditioning procedure. The children were brought into the room with therapists who touched them with cattle prods (sometimes referred to as 'hand held inductoriums'—euphemisms abound in the area) whenever they began to batter themselves. After a few contingent shocks the self-mutilation stopped.

Although successful in treating pathological self-mutilation, shock is virtually useless with problem drinkers. In seeking the correct aversive technique the question to guide the search is: 'given the nature of the problem and its processes, what technique(s) will make contact with these?' The search should begin with the problem and not the technique or some ill-conceived artificial category like 'aversion therapy'. With regard to drinking the specific question is: 'what are the ways to reduce the incentive-expectancy value of alcohol?'

The effects of aversion therapy can be socially embarrassing to the patient

This objection pictures the ex-drinker perpetually on the verge of vomiting the instant he comes within sight or smell of alcohol. Here the term 'aversion therapy' (which for convenience has been used throughout this chapter) is at fault. The effect of pairing a particular drink with a method of inducing nausea is to reduce the incentive value of that substance.[26] Incentive value ('hedonistic tone' is an acceptable substitute) can vary along a continuum from very high to very low. In practice, patients are asked to become familiar with a dimension of incentive value which runs from +10 ('I expect that when I take the drink(s) it will be very, very good') to 0 ('I don't think that it will have an effect on me one way or the other') and is bounded on the lower end by −10 ('I couldn't bear the thought of taking that drink'). Thus the incentive/expectancy rating of a drink can be rated on a 21-point scale. Typically, within five to six pairings the smell and taste ratings move from the neighbourhood of +5 to +9 to around 0 or −2. The verbal descriptions that usually go with these numbers are ones that express indifference, lack of interest or mild distaste. Moreover, if the ratings drop into the −5 to −0 range we have found that they rise up to the 'zone of indifference' (−2 to 0) within a week or two. According to conditioning theory this is a puzzling finding. Changes in the direction opposite to that produced by the pairing are supposed to occur only when the patient has had some outside contact with the alcoholic drink associated with malaise in the clinic ('extinction'). We are at a loss to explain this phenomenon and it is now under study in our laboratory. However, in hundreds of cases we have never observed the incentive ratings to return 'spontaneously' above 0 even months after pairings.

Alcoholics get sick and vomit regularly. Why doesn't that work as a self-cure?

There are two points to be made here. First, actual vomiting, while unpleasant for the moment, actually signals the end of the nausea bout. Drugs like ipecacuana which cause immediate vomiting without nausea are ineffective agents for producing incentive changes. Second, the severe malaise experienced on the morning following drinking is many hours delayed from the act of consumption. (The generalised distress—the hangover, headache and so on—though highly noxious is not at all effective in directly altering the incentive value any more than is electric shock. Once again, it is the quality and not the sheer amount of distress that is the key.) Granted that taste-nausea links are undisturbed by intervals of minutes, it is not clear that any substantial learning can be expected to occur when the delay is in the order of hours. (In our experience, humans show less ability for very long delay conditioning than animals.) For the meantime, the therapist need not be concerned by delays of up to an hour or two: they are known to be safe. Beyond that interval lies uncertainty and probably failure.

You call the procedure 'aversion therapy' and refer to the resulting 'taste aversions', but many alcoholics insist that they 'hate the taste of the stuff'. Why should a taste aversion treatment work if the patient already dislikes the taste of the drink?
It is unfortunate that the terms 'aversion therapy' and 'taste aversion' have come to be used by the scientists who study these procedures. The names will continue to be used, if only to denote areas of research. It is more cumbersome, but more correct, to describe the effects of drink-nausea associations as ones which decrease positive expectancies of and generate neutral-negative visceral changes to that drink (and not to alcohol generally; each type of problem drink must be paired with nausea). The taste as such remains unaffected. It is the expected 'glow' and 'tension reduction' changes brought about by taking alcohol that are altered in a downward direction. 'I don't think I want to have that (i.e. the alcoholic drink) in me' is what the patients often remark after taste aversion therapy. Reports that the drink 'tastes different' are rare.

It is possible to reduce the anticipated attractiveness of alcohol by these methods but once the patient leaves the clinic he will know that he is out of range of the clinician's techniques, on his own and free to drink as he pleases
This objection is a common one and betrays a failure to understand the nature of 'taste-aversion' learning. When a particular substance is ingested and followed each time by a nausea-producing technique, the incentive decline is largely trans-

situational. The effect is non-cognitive and seems to by-pass the mental activities which underpin logic, reasoning and the judgement of circumstance. One famous example was reported by Dr Martin Seligman of the University of Pennsylvania. He went to dinner with his students one evening and, at their suggestion, ordered sauce Bernaise on his meat. The sauce was new to him and he found it delicious. Later on that night, at home, he had a sudden attack of the 'flu, for which he was not entirely unprepared, having felt the symptoms mount over the day. From past experience he knew that severe nausea was a likely part of the symptom cluster. As it turned out, his guess was correct, and he spent the night drifting into and out of a queasy malaise. In a few days he recovered completely and thought no more about the episode until some while later he was given another helping of sauce Bernaise. To his surprise he could not bring himself to eat it. After a moment's reflection he grasped the cause of his change of attitude: not long after eating it on the first occasion he had felt extremely nauseous. Knowing that the nausea was produced by the 'flu and not the food did not change his judgement of the sauce.[27] Where taste and nausea are associated, even if by chance, one might say that 'the head' knows but the stomach does not'.

I had a similar experience many years ago when, with two teenage friends, I deliberately set out to get drunk. We had never done this before and having no idea of the amount required to achieve our goal we purchased a gallon of vermouth. We succeeded in becoming very drunk and, that night and the next morning, violently ill. I can still recall my friend saying the following evening, about his feelings when he woke: 'First I thought I was going to die, then I was afraid I wasn't'. To this day not one of us has touched vermouth. We fully realise that were someone to give us a small glass of vermouth we would be able to restrict our intake to that one glass, but we have found that our rational assessment has no effect on our visceral dislike of the vermouth.

The experimental record with animals and humans is so much in accord with anecdotes such as these that Seligman was led to compare 'taste aversions' with phobias.[28] Both have adaptive value (phobias are usually connected with situations which down the span of time have been a threat to our survival) and neither is susceptible to reversal simply through the provision of valid information ('look, one small glass of vermouth can hardly do you any harm'; or 'a confined space simply cannot hurt you'), ridicule or persuasion. Common to both is the effectiveness of treatment based on graduated exposure. A corollary is that incentive modification therapy will probably not be of any clinical value in patients who are coerced into therapy. A patient given the choice of therapy or jail by the magistrate 'chose' therapy. Aversion therapy was one of the components in the multimodal therapy that we offered in our clinic. The taste-nausea training worked, and it also failed. After ten trials he lost all interest in whisky, the alcohol he drank most often. On the way home, 'cured' but defiant, he purchased a bottle of whisky. He then proceeded to drink his way out of the acquired dislike: he drank, felt ill, had a glass of water, drank some more, felt a little less ill, and so on until he had reversed the process.

Precautions and preparations

As we have emphasised throughout the book, no clinical procedure should be implemented before there is agreement and understanding between patient and therapist. We are particularly careful when using incentive modification to guard against three prevalent misconceptions in the patient: that therapy is a punishment for past misdeeds; that it is a symptom of anger in the therapist; or that he is about to embark on a 100 per cent foolproof cure.

The therapist can avoid reinforcing misconceptions by a careful introduction to the procedures:

> 'The next part of the therapy programme goes by a number of names. You may have heard of it as aversion therapy. The procedure and purpose is simple. By associating the thought, smell and taste of alcohol with something unpleasant it becomes less attractive. From research and clinical cases we know that aversive methods should be ones which produce a degree of nausea (but not vomiting) after you sample the drink. The effect, if we continue for many associations, is to make the expectations of "good feelings" from alcohol much lower. This won't stop you from drinking if you are absolutely determined to do so, but if you do want to stop drinking a certain kind of alcohol the therapy should give you some breathing space and

> the chance to say "no" if somebody tries to press a drink upon you. The therapy won't be pleasant but it isn't dangerous. The way to look at it is that you are being hard on yourself today to be kind on yourself tomorrow.'

This should be followed by a description of how the rotating chair or the covert sensitisation (see below) works. The drinker is given the alcoholic drink to smell and to taste but not to consume and ratings are taken on the +10 to 0 to −10 scale for each trial. The risk of the abstinence-violation effect (and staunch opposition from AA and their allies) if the alcohol is swallowed dictates this strategy. The patient should swish the alcohol around his mouth for 15 seconds and then spit it out into a container supplied for that purpose. When he is securely strapped in the chair it is then revolved at approximately 40 to 50 revolutions per minute. We have found that within five minutes 95 per cent of our large sample rated themselves as 7 or above on a nausea scale of 0 (none) to 10 (unbearable). When this point is reached the trial should be discontinued. It is typical for the nausea ratings to climb a little after the spinning ends. Care should be taken to stop the process before the vomiting (relief) response occurs. After a few minutes, when the patient can again give a zero rating (to avoid a medicinal effect) he should be given the alcoholic drink to smell and taste once again and the routine is run as before. It is important to elicit ratings when and not before the patient reports zero malaise. Otherwise it will be impossible to disentangle conditioned changes from those which merely reflect transient general malaise and the momentary dislike of eating or drinking anything. Three trials per session is the limit we suggest. The procedure is arduous and our wish is not to undermine the patient's motivation to continue.

There is another precaution to be incorporated into incentive modification therapy. The voluminous research into 'taste aversions' has yielded one important law; incentive reductions are more easily formed to novel substances. Familiar foods and fluids can be modified but more trials are needed. However, if a novel substance is consumed at the same time as, or even prior to, consumption the taste of the more familiar substance will be conditioned and the familiar one may not undergo any change. To protect against this possibility we ask patients not to eat or drink anything for two hours before coming to the clinic, especially foods/fluids which are relatively unfamiliar.

Covert sensitisation

If emetic drugs are deemed too risky and resources for constructing a revolving chair are unavailable, covert sensitisation[29] can be employed. In simple terms, covert sensitisation is considered to work exactly as Pavlovian conditioning except that either the to-be-conditioned stimulus (for example, alcohol) and/or the unconditioned stimulus, are presented in a verbal narrative to the patient. Joseph Cautela, who devised the technique, did not question the 'equipotentiality premise'. He believed that the quality of the noxious event made no difference as long as it aroused an aversive response which would, by association, transfer to the alcohol.

Clarke and Hayes[30] looked at the question of the reactions elicited by the verbal stimuli used in covert sentisation. They compared the effects in three groups of volunteers. Each group received the target drink but one had a frightening phobic narrative presented (specially tailored to their phobic sensitivities), another received neutral imagery, while the third was given nausea imagery. Only this group showed declines in the amount consumed and in the incentive ratings given. These findings parallel those from studies using emetic drugs or rotating chairs.

Below are listed representative narratives for covert sensitisation. We have found they work to best effect if the patient sits in a reclining position (eyes closed) and is relaxed or hypnotised. These steps reduce competing and irrelevant thoughts and allow the nausea narrative to achieve full impact. The clinician should read the narrative slowly and adjust it to suit the reactions of the individual patient. As an added modification, 'assisted covert sensitisation' can be employed, with disgusting smells (for example, isobutyric acid) used at crucial times in the narrative.

Scene 1

I'd like you to vividly imagine that you are tasting the fluid that you previously rated. 'See' yourself tasting it, capture the exact taste, colour and consistency. Use all your senses. You are actually drinking it, tasting it, swallowing it, feel the glass in your hand and note the temperature, texture, smell and especially the taste of the fluid.

As you swallow, your stomach starts to churn about and you really feel very sick. You notice a cold sweat breaking out across your back, on your forehead and on the backs of your hands as the nausea increases. The fluid feels unpleasant on your tongue and blocks the back of your throat as your head feels hot and light, slightly headachey, and your eyes refuse to focus properly. You stare at the (beer, whisky, etc.) in the glass, and notice that the odour seems to be increasing your sickness. Thick phlegm gathers at the back of your throat, and you feel as though you might vomit, but you don't get past being on the verge and the sick queasiness remains in the pit of your stomach. What you have swallowed seems to be coagulating in your stomach and throat, refusing to move, slowly choking you, but regardless of your heaving and gagging you cannot vomit, or rid yourself of the taste.

Scene 2

I'd like you to vividly imagine that you are drinking and tasting (beer, whisky, etc.). You are in a (restaurant, pub, etc.) where others are drinking. 'See' yourself there, having a drink. Capture the exact taste of it, the colour and the smell. Use all of your senses. Imagine that you are actually drinking it, tasting it, swallowing it, feel the glass in your hand; and be aware of its temperature, taste and smell, but especially the taste.

As you swallow the drink, a man sitting not far from you gives a low groan, replaces his glass on the table and pushes it away. His head remains lowered as he grasps his stomach with both hands and continues moaning. His eyes are closed now as he grimaces and slowly shakes his head. His face has become a sickly pale colour, and his hands are trembling as he starts to make quick swallowing motions. He opens his eyes and claps both hands over his mouth, but he cannot hold it in and the vomit bursts out. You can see it so clearly. Pieces of food run down his face, soaking his clothes and even reaching the glass. He continues to throw up and particles of his last meal stick to his chin and the hot sticky smell of alcohol reaches you. He really is a disgusting sight. He's got the dry heaves now, there's nothing left to bring up, but his face is still pale and he continues moaning. (Throughout the scene, the appropriate gender references are used according to the composition of the particular group receiving the scene.)

Scene 3
I'd like you to vividly imagine that you are tasting the (beer, whisky, etc.). See yourself tasting it, capture the exact taste, colour and consistency. Use all of your senses. After you've tasted the drink you notice that there is something small and white floating in the glass—it stands out. You bend closer to examine it more carefully, your nose is right over the glass now and the smell fills your nostrils as you remember exactly what the drink tastes like. Now you can see what's in the glass. There are several maggots floating on the surface. As you watch, revolted, one manages to get a grip on the glass and, undulating, creeps up the glass. There are even more of the repulsive creatures in the glass than you first thought. You realise that you have swallowed some of them and you're very aware of the taste in your mouth. You feel very sick and wish that you'd never reached for the glass and had the drink at all.

Summary
Aversion therapy has had a controversial history and has suffered as much from its early defenders as from its later detractors. It is not and never should have been used as the therapy for problem drinking. Equally, detractors have been more emotional than analytical in their objections. Current research supports neither outright rejection nor the unquestioning acceptance of aversive techniques. Today the search should not be for 'the best' aversive techniques but instead should probe for the facets of the problem that may be amenable to incentive modification therapy. Incentive modification is regarded as a way to reduce positive expectancies about the drink paired with nausea. It is best employed where total abstinence is the goal. However, since 'aversions' do not occur to alcohol but rather to the specific tastes used, candidates for controlled drinking who have trouble with certain drinks (for example, who can control their intake of beer but cannot handle spirits) might benefit if those drinks are the target for change.

The research discussed in this chapter is of recent origin but the idea behind it is not. An excellent understanding of aversion therapy for alcoholism appears in the nineteenth century novel by Anne Bronte, *The Tenant of Wildfell Hall*. In the following quotation the heroine gives the details of her method for eliminating the excessive drinking habits of her young son:

'I have succeeded in giving him an absolute disgust for all intoxicating liquors . . . [I] gave him quite as much as his father was accustomed to allow him; as much indeed as he desired to have—but into every glass I surreptitiously introduced a small quantity of tartar-emetic, just enough to produce inevitable nausea and depression without positive sickness. Finding such disagreeable consequences invariably to result from this indulgence he soon grew weary of it . . . When he was thoroughly disgusted with every kind of wine, I allowed him, at his own request to try brandy-and-water, and then gin-and-water . . . I was determined that all should be equally hateful to him. This I have now effected; and since he declares the taste, smell and the sight of any one of them is sufficient to make him sick, I have given up teasing him about them, except . . . as objects of terror in cases of misbehaviour . . . and . . . when he was sick I have obliged the poor child to swallow a little wine-and-water without the tartar emetic . . . because I am determined to enlist all the powers of association in my service . . . I wish this aversion to be so deeply grounded in his nature that nothing in afterlife may be able to overcome it.'

CHAPTER 10

Cognitive Therapy

We will begin this chapter with a hypothetical individual, the ideal patient, seeking help at a treatment centre for an alcohol problem. If the centre is run along modern rather than traditional lines the philosophy of treatment will be expressed in five maxims which will be set out for him by the therapist as follows:

- 'Alcoholism' (a word to be avoided) is not a disease. It is a label used to describe someone who drinks to excess.
- Excessive drinking (a more neutral term) is an acquired set of bad habits.
- These bad habits are linked to maladaptive self-defeating ways of coping with inner and outer pressures.
- Once the self-defeating patterns are identified and their causes are made clear you will be able to learn new and more adaptive coping strategies which do not include the immoderate use of alcohol.
- Problems in your social, occupational or marital life may be highly correlated with excessive drinking but they do not directly cause it.

Our ideal patient will then join with the therapist in a detailed search for the high-risk antecedents, the emotional states and the consequences of drinking which serve to maintain destructive drinking habits. Diligent work in recording each drink, and faithful compliance with all of the other 'homework' requests made of him (plus the understanding cooperation of his spouse, if he is married) will set the stage for the remaining steps in therapy. The regular, correct use of the appropriate self-control behaviours (relaxation, meditation, assertive behaviour and others) will bring drinking and the associated problems to an end and therapy to a satisfactory and permanent conclusion. So it would go with the ideal patient.

Next we can consider the reactions of a real patient, Patient

Two. After many years of drinking he has come to therapy reluctantly and with mixed motives. He harbours fears about the effects of his drinking, fears which he may have held for some time, but it is some sort of crisis—medical, mental or occupational—that has supplied the impetus for him to seek treatment. In contrast with Patient One's receptivity, this man begins his interactions with the therapist committed to certain beliefs about why he has alcohol problems and holds a set of expectancies about what must be done to effect a 'cure'. The probability that, at the start of therapy, there will be a commonality of views on these critical issues between him and the therapist is not high. From the therapist's side of the desk the patient is likely to appear stubborn, antagonistic and uncooperative.

Cognitive and behavioural writings have given little attention to patients who do not automatically cooperate with suggestions and directions and treatments given 'for their own good'. Traditional treatments do at least recognise that therapist-patient difficulties are the rule and not the exception. Where we part company with orthodox practitioners is on the reasons for disagreements, drop-outs and failures. The usual accusations of 'poor motivation' and 'denial' are tactics of blame and not explanation. Such charges do nothing to promote conciliation and direct attention away from the critical interactions following preliminary contact.

In Chapter 5 we discussed the establishment of trust in the first interview, emphasising the necessity for courtesy and the assurance of confidentiality. Working on the probability that the whole rationale of cognitive therapy will be novel to most patients, we follow the first interview with what we call rationale therapy, with the aim of establishing a commonality of outlook between patient and therapist. Its omission sets the stage for failure.

The reasons why failures occur are many, but our impression is that the blame lies in the 'tabula rasa' assumption which is too often the starting point in the cognitive-behavioural therapist's thinking about the patient. The patient is taken to have no set views and it is thought that he will improve if the correct therapies are given. Experimentally-oriented clinicians are likely to take care in gathering all-important assessments regarding the amounts and frequency of drinking, dependence levels, associated problems and the rest. What can be overlooked is the patient's 'theory' of his problems. This results in a failure to obtain a clear picture of his ideas, and especially his reactions to the therapist's requests and rationales. When reading cognitive-behavioural manuals one is struck by the assumption that the patient is a willing partner who will do all that he is 'requested to carry out', 'asked to record' and 'reminded to do'. Therapy is presented as moving in one direction only, with the main job of the therapist being to impart facts as the basis for developing treatment programmes. If facts by themselves could uproot beliefs then our caveats and, along with them, our emphasis on rationale therapy and cognitive restructuring could be dismissed as superfluous. However, taking a useful finding from an experiment reported in a technical journal is one thing; persuading the patient to alter his views on the basis of data alone is entirely another.

Cognitive therapy: overview and rationale

The principle conceptual and treatment influences to emerge in the last decade directed at attitude as well as behaviour change have come from the cognitive model of emotions and behaviour. It is associated with the names of Ellis, Lazarus, Beck and Meichenbaum. Later we will take up some of the distinctions amongst them in their respective therapies (especially Ellis) but first the many points of agreement. In applying the cognitive models to drinking problems we begin with the assumption that the problem drinker will have to deal with emotional stresses and difficulties within himself and in his relations with others. A neat distinction cannot be drawn between inter- and intra-personal difficulties: each creates stress reactions and attempts at coping, often misdirected. In therapy the coping strategies taught are primarily attempts (a) to control emotional distress through the application of new interpretations and other cognitive manoeuvres and (b) to equip the patient to cope with external pressures which originate in his social life. Following customary usage we will discuss the first under the heading cognitive restructuring and for the second we will use the term interpersonal coping strategies. The starting point for both is cognition and cognitive therapy. First, we will give a brief outline of the 'cognitive therapy' and then give a cognitive-behavioural orientation to alcohol problems.

To begin, cognitive therapies emphasise the distinctions between cognition, feeling and action. Most clinicians routinely search for feeling (mood) and behaviour disorders in their interactions with problem drinkers, but the word 'cognition' may still be more familiar to the researcher than the clinical practitioner. Very generally, the word 'cognition' covers the activities of language, judgement and the psychological systems underlying the behaviours of planning, goal setting and choosing amongst alternatives. This is a partial list, but it suggests the processes in which cognitions are minimally involved, such as inborn reflexes, automatic adjustments to change in posture, the knee-jerk reaction startle and sneezing; all such reactions, and others like them, can be thought of as 'stimulus-bound' reactions. They are prop erly classified as re-actions because their appearance and magnitude is determined by the presence and intensity of the eliciting stimulus. When the 'drive' stimuli are removed the reflexive responses terminate. Learning, habit and upbringing play, at most, a small part in shaping the form and maintenance of these responses.

Both cognitive and reflexive activities involve the brain and complex mental circuitry operate in both. Thus the difference we are aiming at is not captured in the difference between 'simple' and 'complex'. We find Hebb's[1] definition and distinction the most useful: cognitions are conceived of as 'subject-directed, semi-autonomous ['mental'] activities'. The operations of cognition, which are heavily based on past experience, form the basis of planning, expectations, judgements and evalutions that we make of ourselves and others. Interactions are possible between reflexive and cognitive systems. One may decide beforehand, say for a substantial amount of money, to leave one's hand on a hot stove and endure the pain. Similarly, a sudden sneeze or startle reflex may be interpreted cognitively as an embarrassing faux pas. Nevertheless, there is a fundamental distinction beween cognitive and reflexive systems which will feature prominently in the treatment of alcohol problems: the cognitive systems of evaluation, judgement, planning (faulty or adaptive) are not 'forced' by the contextual circumstances in which they occur. Hebb's term 'semi-autonomous' conveys this important idea—that there is potential (though perhaps unrealised) freedom to alter for the better cognitive reactions and the emotional states they can produce, even if the external circumstances in which they take place remain unchanged.

Intermediate between cognitive and reflexive are classically conditioned reactions. These are formed by the pairing of a neutral event, the to-be-conditioned stimulus (CS) with a biologically powerful event, the unconditioned stimulus (UCS). Thus a tone for Pavlov's dogs, because it was followed by food, triggered a salivation response. Pavlovian reactions have also been recorded in humans. One provocative experiment pertinent to understanding alcohol disorders was a demonstration that the smell (CS) of alcohol provoked cravings and salivation in drinkers receiving treatment.[2] These responses are not 'cognitive' in the sense that we are using the word. For now the best way to state the difference is that classically conditioned reactions are closer to reflexive than cognitive in their 'slave-like' tie to the evoking circumstances.

The interactions of classically conditioned reactions and the 'higher mental process' of cognitions are not completely understood. Words as well as other stimuli can become conditioned stimuli, and, in the other direction, with training, inner talk can inhibit or diminish classically conditioned reactions. The consensus would be that cognitions are extremely important in understanding the psychology of alcohol problems, especially in the initiation of drinking bouts. We know now that they play a central role in the treatment of interpersonal stressors. There are numerous recent reports revealing a strong link between uncontrolled drinking and 'negative emotional states'[3] which support this contention.

Misinformation and faulty beliefs are the two forms of maladaptive cognitions which appear time and again in the all-important early stages of (rationale) therapy.

Misinformation in particular must not be overlooked: there are many who, at great cost to their well-being, completely subscribe to the mistaken ideas outlined in Chapter 1. Faulty information is easily corrected. The same is not true of faulty beliefs. Two different types of beliefs appear regularly and are best dealt with in the following sequence. First there are erroneous beliefs of a general nature about the causes of negative emotions which say that the things, events and people in one's world are the direct causes of our emotional life ('he made me mad'). The second type of cognitive error is based on the erroneous belief that one's emotional happiness depends upon oneself and others adhering to rules which are couched in the form of 'shoulds' and 'oughts' (for example, 'I should be the centre of attention'; 'I ought to retaliate to every criticism').

There are three parts to rationale therapy. Initially, with the minimum of good advice, the patient's 'world view' should be elicited: that is his reasons for seeking help, his belief in the need for and possibility of change and the means of achieving it. The second part requires the therapist to give *his* perspective on the problem, to present in nontechnical language the bases in the evidence for his position, to outline the possible goals in therapy and to clarify the nature of the relationship between the two participants in the therapeutic transaction. In the final and most difficult part the theories and techniques of cognitive behaviour therapy must be translated into the patient's language and thus into practice. If these vital matters are neglected, potentially effective techniques, though firmly anchored in data, may seem silly and irrelevant to the patient. Through examples, vignettes, Socratic dialogue and informal experiments the patient must be helped to see the point of the suggested techniques.

To begin, there are certain key questions which can give the therapist insight into how easy or difficult the days ahead promise to be. The first of these is the simple request 'Why are you here now?' or 'What is the main reason for seeking help at this point in your life?' As a means of highlighting the potential complications we will take two patients, Mr A and Mr Z, who have identical drinking histories, consume roughly the same, excessive amount of alcohol each day and score at precisely the same levels on a test of dependence. Mr A, no less than Mr Z, suffers from serious bouts of anger, depression and remorse in connection with his drinking. The clinician can be reasonably sure from the intake assessment data that both men are at the threshold of serious disorders in all areas of their lives.

To the unenquiring clinician in both cases the reasons for the men entering therapy may appear self-evident. The list of disorders is so imposing the only wonder is that Messrs A and Z have waited so long before seeking help. It is, however, a serious mistake to proceed directly to interview-assessment procedures before gaining an insight into the patients' beliefs. Let us contemplate the costs of that path of action.

Suppose it were the case that Mr A realises that his drinking has something to do with his response each day to pressures to have just 'a few' after work and perhaps with certain marital tensions. Mr Z's self-assessment differs considerably. Unlike Mr A, he is blind to his own part in perpetuating his troubles. In seeking answers he may alternate between attributing his drinking to an inherited disease and the other extreme of blaming the nightly battles with his wife who he says upsets him and drives him to drink. Mr A believes that with the right assistance he can learn to take control over his drinking; Mr Z believes that he is powerless to stop until his wife 'stops making him angry', or until a doctor steps in, takes charge and does 'something medical'.

For a Mr A the clinician can proceed directly to the skills acquisition and application stages which are discussed later and in the remaining chapters. We all hope for patients like Mr A but the fact is that therapists can expect to encounter a steady flow of patients who, to a greater or lesser extent, resemble the hypothetical Mr Z. Questions which can be used in the early stages to obtain an insight into the patient's attitudes but are often left out of interview schedules are:

1. Have you been in therapy before? (If the answer is 'yes' ask the following two questions.)
2. Why did you leave? (The patient's reasons can provide valuable clues to his motivations, for example 'we couldn't get along,' or 'it took too long,' or 'he never really listened to me,' or 'he said I was an alcoholic'.)
3. What did you do in therapy? (If the therapist used one form of 'relaxation' and it failed, the patient can be taught another, more effective method [see Chapter 11], the differences can be explained and the patient's cooperation restored.)

If the replies suggest that there have been past failures that arose out of a clash of beliefs then special care must be taken when outlining the cognitive position before proceeding to the next stage.

The cognitive-behavioural orientation

Before a Mr Z can enter into the therapeutic process he must undergo a 'paradigm shift', a wholesale reorientation to the actual as opposed to the apparent causes of his problems. Patients like Mr Z see themselves as helpless, driven by a collection of causes over which they have no control. We can call this the 'puppet theory' of personality and behaviour. Or, in a different language, we could say that Mr Z has, unwittingly, given his unreserved commitment to a stimulus (S) response (R) theory of thinking, feeling and behaving. Though he may not know it, this theory was once, thirty or more years ago, the leading behavioural explanation of all behaviour. It said, in essence, present the S and the R will appear, the 'glue' that holds them together being habit training (as supplied in our culture in its daily round of activities).

Since that time ideas about emotions and behaviour have undergone a radical change and growth in sophistication. It is the therapist's job to make Mr Z aware of the changes, not just as a shift in academic thinking but as a fundamental redirection in the meaning we assign to drinking problems and their amelioration.

The application of cognitive-behaviour therapy: challenging maladaptive beliefs about cognitions, emotions and causality

Experiments, case studies and surveys have established that excessive drinking before therapy, backsliding during it, and relapses afterwards are closely correlated with interpersonal discord.[4] Sanchez-Craig et al.'s[5] subjects listed alcohol as a way of coping with stressful situations in 90 per cent of the drinking episodes described. The emotions most often cited were depression, anger, fear and anxiety. Similar findings were uncovered by Littman and her team.[6] What drinkers do not see and are slow to accept is that they have a responsibility for their emotional reactions as they are more closely related to their cognitions than to the behaviour of others. To the patient it will seem implausible that 'mere thoughts' can generate negative emotions. It is even harder to bring him around to accept that, in point of fact, no one can make him angry (depressed, anxious, frustrated, violent, etc.). The message the therapist has to deliver in a convincing way is that it is not the angry words of others but the significance the patient gives to them that is the cause of emotional distress, counter attacks and drinking bouts. When a patient reports that his wife's 'nagging' depressed and angered him and drove him to drink, he is embracing errors both of causality and of the 'shoulds and oughts' variety: (a) 'she made me angry'; (b) 'people shouldn't criticise me,' and (c) 'when someone has made me feel bad I have to drink'.

The therapist's task in cognitive restructuring is twofold. With soft arguments and telling examples he has to convince the patient that he is making a causal statement, of which he may well be unaware, and that he imagines, incorrectly, that his emotions have the character of a reflex response. Just as the knee jerks when the doctor taps it with his rubber hammer, the patient is in effect stating that he is 'jerked' into a state of anger (or some other distress) by his wife's critical words (or by an experience of failure, disappointments, etc.).

Once the patient understands that other and more positive emotional and behavioural reactions are possible in these same circumstances the self-defeating shoulds and oughts can be challenged and the patient introduced to the all-important distinction between events which are correlated with one another and events which are the adequate and direct causes of a particular reaction. Simple, homely examples will serve this purpose. To give the flavour, two are outlined here:

> 'I am going to say something now which may put us in immediate disagreement. My claim is that your wife didn't make you angry yesterday evening. More than that, neither she nor anyone else has ever made you or could make you angry. I realise this appears to contradict the obvious, but I'll try to convince you that my statement is neither silly or outrageous. Let me start with this example. Suppose I were to drop my pen on the floor and, suppose further, an instant later someone were to knock on my door. It would not be reasonable to say that by dropping the pen I caused (i.e. made) someone knock on the door. The two events are correlated but not caused by each other. Here is another example. Suppose at 2 p.m. one day while working at my desk an angry colleague knocked at my door, walked in, proceeded to abuse me for five minutes, then left. Had I got angry (or depressed, or whatever), would it not seem reasonable to say that his outburst caused my anger? After all, at 1.59 I had been working in a happy frame of mind (fact one). At 2.00 he knocked at the door (fact two). When he left at 2.05 I was agitated and angry (fact three). Thus far we have three facts, all of which could be verified by unbiased onlookers. But try to see that I make a mistake if I turn a given fact (fact two) into the cause of my anger (fact three). To repeat, I am not contesting any of the facts. We can agree on them with-

out argument. But let us look at my anger. Anger is a word for a collection of changes in the body and the mind: typically, blood pressure climbs, respiration rate increases, levels of physical tension climb, the heart beats faster and hostile thoughts cross my mind. Let us take a few parts of this collection of mental and physical reactions that we have just summarised with the one word "anger". When I become angry I clench my jaw. Who actually clenches it? The answer is "I do". My colleague doesn't rush over and hold my jaw to create this tension. Now let us take some of my mental reactions which were active then: "Who does he think he is? . . . That was damn rude and unfair of him." (And if I have lost all self control) "I'll fix him!" Now, did he put those thoughts in my brain? Again, the answer is "No". Did he make me breathe faster? "No." All of these were my own reactions. Notice I am not saying that he was right or wrong in what he said. Nor did I say that I should surrender to his point of view. What I am saying is that the turmoil (not the disagreement) is my responsibility. I am also saying that disagreement does not automatically—does not have to—generate emotional turmoil. Granted the two often do go together, as we know. The question, and challenge, is, do they *have* to? The evidence says no.[7]

The same holds true for the "nagging": it did not *make* you drink. I realise that you often drink heavily under such circumstances (many do), but you were not compelled to fetch the bottle of whisky, take a glass and drink yourself blind.'

In one instance a man with some training in anatomy and psychology contested my reinterpretation. When I said that his wife's badgering did not (a) make him angry and (b) was not the cause of his drinking, he replied, 'Oh yes it was. The stimuli of her voice and the sight of her angry face were processed in the auditory and visual channels, went up to the thalamus and on to the upper-brain and from there down to the emotional centres and [his explanation for the drinking] to the motor centres.' My reply, which was successful, was put together in haste and a touch of resignation, for he was particularly resistant to my arguments:

'Let's imagine you are in your car with me beside you. The traffic lights are red. You are waiting for the lights to turn green so that you can continue with your journey. But before they do I offer to give you $10 000 if, when they turn green, you stay exactly where you are. Granted you'll receive a good deal of angry looks as cars pass around you. If you stay there long enough a member of the police will come along and fine you. Suppose the fine is $100: your net gain will be $9900. Now, here is the point of this little story. When lights turn from red to green you take your foot from the brake and place it on the accelerator. You've done this thousands of times, as do all other drivers. But the visual stimulus of the green light did not lift your foot from the brake to the accelerator. You chose to do it, as my example proved. Granted, through "force of habit" you may do it in an automatic, machine-like fashion. However, if you become aware of your ability to select other options, then you can "de-automatise". This applies to your emotions and your decisions to drink. You have more freedom than you imagine.'

RET, ABC and Albert Ellis

One of the founders of cognitive therapy, Albert Ellis, coined the term rational-emotive therapy (RET). The words indicate the supposed direction of influence, from cognitive activities to affective reactions. We may take issue with the idea that all negative affect is the direct result of maladaptive (Ellis calls them 'irrational') beliefs and negative self-talk. The evidence to which he refers is correlational and does not provide a basis for making causal statements. Supporters point out that depressed individuals and excessive drinkers endorse more negative statements and exhibit significantly more self deprecation than 'normals'.[8] One interpretation is that given by Ellis: bad thoughts → irrational beliefs → bad feelings. There is substance to this claim but there is evidence that affect can precede as well as follow cognition through any one of a number of pathways.[9] In either case RET can be employed to control and reduce maladaptive emotional reactions.

The process of rationale therapy as outlined thus far is well illustrated by Ellis's ABC technique. 'A' stands for the situation (for example, being criticised), 'B' for the patient's interpretation and 'C' for his emotional reactions. Patients are painfully aware of C, the emotional disturbance, but usually put the blame for it on A—events, people or situations. Thus A-C connections are what they perceive, and they can conceive of but three strategies for alleviating emotional distress: avoid A; placate (or dominate) A; or, barring that, take the 'medication' (alcohol) to block the response systems underlying C (and,as is known, such relief is short-lived at best). Cognitive therapy hinges on the patient acknowledging the existence and importance of B (thoughts, beliefs, self-statements) and it may require many examples and repetitions before the point is grasped. Here is an example of how Ellis's ABC technique can be used in the rationale stage:

Therapist: Look, you say that ridicule makes you drink, which is another way of saying that A (the ridicule) causes C (the anxiety). OK, let's have a look at that. If you encounter ridicule, A, but immediately following that you remember a friendly reaction earlier from someone you really like, what happens?

Patient: It doesn't bother me as much; maybe not at all.

Therapist: Well, that's interesting, because what we have here are identical A's but two different emotional reactions:

A1 (ridicule)	C1 (brood, get drunk)
A2 (ridicule)	C2 (indifference to ridicule)

Notice that A1 is identical to A2 but C2 is very different from C1. How come? Isn't it possible that between the 'ridicule' and your hurt feelings something important is going on in the way you size up things? We'll call that something the B part, which now give us A–|B→B sequence. The barrier line between A and B and the arrow from B to C are meant to indicate where the real causal relation exists.'

If all the examples leave the drinker unconvinced, then his objections must be sought and answered. The typical ones are:

Objection 1: Emotion is a part of life: what you're saying is that I should be cold and unfeeling.

Reply: Nothing of the sort. There are many pleasant emotions like love, joy, playfulness and humour, which enrich our lives. What I've been trying to say is that the negative triad of anxiety, anger and depression are self-caused, self-defeating, get in the way of solving problems and prompt you to drink.

Objection 2: (sarcastically) Oh, I'm supposed to feel really happy when somebody attacks me:

Reply: By no means. If you feel that you're right, say so, but depression or anger will not make your position any more correct or convince the other person of the 'error of his ways'.

Objection 3: Some emotions are inevitable. If my best friend dies I'm going to feel really bad.

Reply: Yes, I agree. And it would be understandable for you to feel that way. But if negative emotions persist for days, weeks or months, then you are subjecting yourself to extremes of distress which do you no good (nor your deceased friend) and if it continues, given your past history, you're likely to get into trouble with alcohol.

Objection 4: But it's better (that is, psychologically healthier) to get rid of the anger than to keep it 'all bottled up inside'.

Reply: There is something in what you say. A clinical researcher, Alan Marlatt, and his colleagues put volunteers in situations where confederates of the investigators deliberately insulted them. The angry ones who got a chance to retaliate (giving shocks in a later 'experiment') were less stressed than those who did not get that opportunity. So once you have lost your poise and sense of control maybe it is better to express anger, but you do not have to lose control in the first place. Later on we'll look at ways to express disagreement openly but without anger.

Objection 5: OK, maybe what you say is right in theory, but in ordinary life people can't expect to live lives free of worry, anxiety and your other 'negative emotions'.

Reply: Again, I agree. The assumptions and interpretations which give rise to destructive feelings and drinking can happen so quickly that before you know it you've blown your top once more or slipped into depression. That's probably true of everybody to some extent. But ask yourself: 'for how long need it last?' If you practice awareness and 'owning your own emotions' you can reduce the duration of the slip, and even more substantially still as you practice cognitive therapy.

Objection 6: Yes, now it does make sense. But how do I change? You say it's the evaluations and interpretations of B that make the difference. But I'm not aware of my Bs. Everything goes so fast and before I know it I'm upset and into the booze.

Reply: You've put your finger on a very important problem. The B activities become so well learned that they seem to operate out of our consciousness. Take this example. [I show the patient the sequence /-\ I3 C I) and ask him to read it quickly. The symbols are always read by patients as four letters of the alphabet. Then below it I write 11 12 13 14 15, cover up the first sequence and ask them to read the second sequence aloud. All patients read these symbols as numerals. Then I point to the similarity of B in the letter sequence to 13 in the number sequence.] Now you called the first one B and the second 13. But it could have been A I3 C D or conversely 11 12 B 14 15 etc. or A 1 3 and so on. I did not say letters in the first case, nor did I say numerals in the second. The 13 was your interpretation of what I wanted of you but it was not a deliberate, conscious one. In answer to your question 'how do I change?' we must expand the ABC formula to include D for disputation. Later on I'll give you some forms to fill out to help you with the process [see Appendix C]. An extra aid is the boy scout motto: 'Be Prepared'. Think ahead to situations which have given you trouble and plan what you will do well beforehand instead of slipping into the usual self-defeating habits of getting upset or giving in to pressure and drinking out of control. We'll cover these when we discuss relapse therapy.

Objection 7: When and how much I drink has got nothing to do with who is with me, friendly or not, nor the time of day nor what I am thinking.

Reply: While it may feel that you get urges to drink which come from out of the blue these desires, however they begin, do not force you to go to the bottle shop nor are the 'urges' or 'cravings' the same thing as actually taking that first drink. The 'urge' (to drink) is not the same as the 'act' (of drinking). However, if you believe that they are, then the desire for a drink will soon be followed by your drinking a second, a third and so on. Second, though it may not be easy to see it, if you look closely there will be connections between certain things that happen to you and the desire to drink. What I'd like you to do is record any urges you have in the following week on a 1–100 scale (low urges being numbered 1, 2, 3 and so on, with, say, 95 indicating a very strong desire) and where they occur. When people do this they usually find that it is an unpleasant emotional state which precedes the urge or seeing someone having a drink or smelling a drink that awakens an urge. [In the case of the latter, 'extinction therapy' may be used in conjunction with cognitive therapy. This is discussed in Chapter 12.] Even in highly dependent individuals, drinking will not be completely free of situational influences, interpretations made about them, and decisions to drink (or to drink to excess). The effective use of the cognitive therapies depends upon the patient realising this.

The cognitive therapies of Beck can make a useful complement to Ellis's emphasis on 'irrational beliefs'. Beck has written little about drinking problems but his ideas can be applied in this area. In these pages we can give no more than a short outline of his work: for further details see Beck's book on cognitive therapy.[10] The basic ideas are that we can develop maladaptive schemas which bias and distort our recall of critical events. Patients fall into arbitrary inferences, selective perceptions (emphasis of the negative and diminution of the positive) and overgeneralisations. Therapy consists of challenges in the form of 'experiments' that the patient carries out to test his perceptions. In so doing he uses his data to discover his distortions and through this comes to the realisation that he is in charge of his own depression and anxiety.

Implementation outside the clinic

With the preceding rationale therapy as a basis, the patient is ready to enter the action stages of therapy, the behavioural phase of cognitive-behaviour therapy. As a prelude, the therapist should sketch out the model which will guide the interactions between him and his patient. This preamble should include a simple account of the evidence against 'loss of control' and the 'disease theory' of alcoholism. The modest genetic influence can be acknowledged without slipping into a counsel of despair. While the genetic evidence does not favour the inevitability of alcoholism, it should alert the patient to the fact that he must take more care than those without any such vulnerability. This is a variant of Meehl's stress-diathesis account.[11] In these early talks the goals of controlled drinking and total abstinence (in connection with high dependence) can be covered. At every stage special care should be taken to enlist the patient's active cooperation. The relationship should be implicitly and openly signalled as collaborative, psychoeducational, skill-focussed and present-centred. The past may feature but only insofar as it brings into clear view the recurrent patterns and high-risk situations of the present. For cognitive-behavioural therapies the here-and-now is the testing place for therapy; long searches into the distant past in quest of 'the origins' are given low priority.

The advice and techniques at this early stage can be applied whether controlled drinking or abstinence is the treatment goal. First of all the patient is introduced to the basic aims of the programme:

- To pinpoint the situations in which drinking goes beyond reasonable limits.
- To draw inferences about the evaluative, attitudinal, interpretive (i.e. B) responses to these situations.
- To identify the emotional distress experienced (such as depression or anger).
- To learn the inter- and intra-personal skills which will maintain reasonable drinking (or abstinence).

A part of the 'housekeeping' duties of the early meetings is reaching agreement as to the maximum number of sessions which should pass before progress (if any) is evaluated and new directions are contemplated. The patient must agree that regular attendance and/or adequate notification of any cancellation is required. Another condition for beginning work together is that the patient must not take any alcohol before coming to a session.

The next step is to request a period of complete abstinence. Sanchez-Craig's (personal communication) rationale is simple, persuasive and to the point:

> 'Regular heavy use of alcohol for five or more years tends to dull people's cognitive abilities. Heavy drinkers often lose part of their capacity to abstract, to solve problems and to learn new things. . . . [R]esearch has shown that if drinkers with characteristics similar to yours abstain [or take no more than one standard drink a day] then intellectual abilities sharpen again. Since the program requires skill learning and problem solving, two to three weeks of abstinence will help you to learn more efficiently.
>
> When heavy drinkers attempt to abstain, they usually experience two types of difficulties: their own temptations to drink and pressures from others. . . . A period of abstinence . . . can give you an opportunity to observe how you cope spontaneously [in such circumstances].'

This rationale is, obviously, only appropriate for those who are going to work towards controlled drinking. For the heavily dependent drinker or those for whom abstinence is mandated, suitable modifications emphasising progress towards complete avoidance are advised. In either case the patient can agree to work towards this goal by stopping that day or by tapering off. If the decision is to taper off then a contract should be written and agreed to, specifying how quickly the reduction is to occur and under what circumstances (for example, reduction of one standard drink each day; no drinking at lunch hour). The therapist should take the lead in suggesting the rate of decline in drinks per day. He is also advised to get expectancy ratings from the patient. The scale for measuring these can run from 'very confident' through 'confident' and 'slightly confident' to 'not confident at all'. If the likely success of suggestions for change is rated in the latter two categories it might be as well to ask the patient to set up a tapering off programme in which he can feel 'very confident'.

Self-monitoring

The initial assessments to obtain a picture of drinking history, estimates of recent levels of consumption and dependence levels are all based upon the patient's recall of facts in the recent and distant past. Self-monitoring is connected to present treatment goals. It is to be carried out on a daily basis because retrospective recordings are known to be unreliable.[12] Self-monitoring goes beyond mere drink counting: it includes a description of context and high-risk situations and the emotional responses connected to drinking. The rationale should be presented by the therapist to the patient in this sort of way:

> 'During the coming week if you drink any alcohol I would like you to list when, with whom and where you drank [controlled drinkers should note whether pre-set limits were exceeded], your companions' reactions, your evaluations, emotional reactions and actions (left the room, had a few, etc.) Self-monitoring is boring and arduous, but necessary. If your memory is like mine then trying to recall the details of last Thursday will prove impossible. So do this each day and try to stick with it. Daily self-monitoring is the only way we can detect patterns. Self-recording is essential also for monitoring progress towards our goals. Another benefit is that you might

find that when you actually carry it out you become aware of certain drinking patterns which are more or less automatic.'

For those whose goal is abstinence the request to self-monitor could seem to amount to a prediction of failure by the therapist ('I don't intend to drink; I told him so and yet he asks me to record all my drinks. Doesn't he believe me?') Left unremarked, this could precipitate a break in the relationship. A few words of reassurance should settle the patient's doubts.

> 'When I ask you to record drinks consumed and the rest of the related details, please do not think that I am assuming that you will drink (or drink to excess). If a day passes and you do not drink, fine, record a zero, but if you do have a slip be sure to record that too. Your actions, the type of drink, the amount you consumed and under what conditions, and crucial cognitions and emotions can provide us with valuable clues as to where the trouble spots are.'

It should be stressed to the patient that retrospective recording is of little use, and therefore a self-monitoring diary should be kept every day without fail. The patient should be asked to bring in his diary each session. It can serve as a basis for planning the subsequent week's work.

Involving the spouse

At an early stage we ask the patient's permission to interview his spouse or partner. (Although the gap between male and female problem drinkers is narrowing, the patient is still more likely to be male. The spouse/partner is therefore here taken to be female.) The spouse may not come, and if she does, she may have significant distortions in her own estimation of the patient's drinking problems. As with the patient, the therapist should refrain from intruding too formal a structure at the start. Gradually he can lead into a general history taking (especially of drinking or other drug problems in close relatives), discussion of marital adjustment (does she see the situation as hopeless or can she envisage improvement?), and enquire as to the reactions of the children to their father's drinking problem.

Before gathering data on the wife's view of the evolution of the drinking problem and its current status, it is worth stating again that the therapist must be on guard against distortions in her account. If there is a wide disparity between the patient's self-recordings of drinking and his wife's estimates over the same period, then an impasse will result until the therapist can uncover the reasons for it. Explaining the notion of the 'standard drink' to the wife might settle the issue. Where a disagreement continues, the therapist can suggest that the client and his wife compare recording sheets on a day-to-day basis. Diplomacy is essential and the therapist, above all, must avoid taking sides or, worse, sitting as a judge delivering a verdict. The difficulty may lie in the wife's belief that drinking is an unvarying response, whereas in fact, it fluctuates markedly with circumstances.

As a last resort the therapist can ask the patient if he would agree to random home visits to be given a breathalyser test. This suggestion is far from ideal: the patient may feel he is on trial or even that the therapist does not believe him. Some attempt should be made to quiet these fears: 'Between your estimates and your wife's there is a considerable gap. One of you seems to be getting it wrong. Would you mind if on certain evenings I phone you (to make sure you don't have visitors) and come over with a breathalyser in order to get a quick reading?' If the patient disagrees then the issue of drink assessment should be pursued further. Some clinicians would take issue with our recommendations, considering home visits as intrusive and counter-productive: for them therapy is an encounter that occurs within the confines of the office and the 50-minute hour. Clearly we are out of sympathy with this attitude.

Finally, the therapist should cover with the spouse the same ground as was covered with the patient (genetic factors, stress diathesis, the nexus between drinking and family strife, the concept of dependence and the notion of high risk situations).

If the couple has been in therapy before they might well have heard the wife blamed for the spouse's drinking. Popular theory says that a wife wishes to keep her husband locked into his drinking problems, thus satisfying her neurotic needs for control. He fulfils these by unconsciously agreeing to play the role of problem drinker. Whalen[13] described four types of wives of heavy drinkers. The first is 'Suffering Susan' who has a need for punishment and seeks out a partner who will satisfy her wishes. The second type he describes as 'Controlling Catherine', who chooses a weak husband to give her pathological need for dominance full play. 'Wavering Winnie needs affection and selects an affectionate alcoholic spouse, and 'Punitive Polly' is (selfishly) career-centred and aggressive. He produces no evidence whatever for these assertions. Perhaps there are some women who seek out men who are problem drinkers and either attempt to reform them or enjoy the solicitous concern they receive from others. For the majority reality is very different from this stereotype. As Edwards remarks: 'cruel mistakes result from being persuaded that this is the picture of the alcoholic marriage. . . . For . . . the truth of the matter is that when the husband begins to drink excessively the wife inevitably then has to make the choice between letting the house go to rack and ruin or taking much of its running into her own hands; it can be seen, then, that dominance is merely adjustive'.[14] Most telling of all, when problem drinkers bring their drinking under control, the mental state of their partner improves. If the neurotic wife theory were correct, then it would be expected that as her husband improved she would begin a period of psychological deterioration. Wives of problem drinkers improve psychologically when they are away from them. Griffith gives these figures: 82 per cent of the wives reported strong symptoms of distress while the husband was drinking and 43 per cent when he attained sobriety. A careful review of the literature reveals that the wives of problem drinkers possess normal basic personalities.[15]

Intrapersonal techniques: assertiveness

'Come on George, have one (or one more) with us; don't be a spoilsport,' say his friends. He replies: 'No thanks, I'm cutting down (or knocking off) for health reasons, but go ahead and enjoy yourselves. Don't let me stop you." The opening sentence is an example of the pressure to drink, or to drink excessively. Pressure from others to take alcohol is second only to negative emotions as a precipitate of drinking, excessive drinking and relapse. George's behaviour was a model of assertiveness. What is uncommon about the episode is the ease with which George maintained his own wishes, cordially but firmly, when put under pressure to do otherwise. No abstinence or controlled drinking programme can be considered complete if assertiveness therapy has not been included.

What is assertiveness? Definitions and, accordingly, therapies differ. We have seen it listed as:

1. minimal aggressivesness;
2. a way to acquire reinforcers or rewards;
3. the unrestrained expression of feelings;
4. standing up for your rights;
5. communicating sensibly, without undue emotion, where there are differences of outlook.

The first definition can be dismissed: even if aggressiveness gains the sought-after reward, the cost to interpersonal relationships outweighs the momentary gain. The second, which says that one's emotional wellbeing rests entirely in the hands of others and the rewards they care to dispense, is not only misconceived but encourages people to try to change or blame others rather than to develop the skills of self-regulation. The third has a place if the feelings are expressed honestly and tactfully: there is no evidence that unreflective over-emoting accomplishes anything useful. The 'standing up for your rights' definition suggests an adversarial attitude instead of one based on mutual understanding. We favour the fifth, which is taken from Lange and Jacubowski's very useful manual on assertiveness. Our own definition is closest to theirs: assertiveness is another name for tactful truth telling. Though it sounds reasonable it has the one fault of making assertiveness sound easy.

People do not find assertiveness in any of its forms easy (saying 'No' to a request; asking a favour 'Look, when we get to the party don't keep asking me to have a drink'; accepting a compliment, etc.). Why is this so? Two rival answers are currently popular. The first is known as the 'skills deficit model', and says that people are unassertive and succumb to pressure because the relevant interpersonal skills to resist are absent from their behavioural repertoire. If so steps should be taken to rectify the deficit by training people in these skills. Proponents of this position often use the term 'assertion training' which carries the implication that, like the novice driver, the unassertive patient must be taught the skills by an instructor, and then go on to practice and perfect them.

The major rival to the skills deficit model is the 'response inhibition model'. This says that in most situations involving drinking people already possess the skills (if it makes sense to think of the timely phrase 'no more for me thanks' as a skill) but are afraid of being evaluated negatively by others. Thus a major problem is anxiety associated with the possibility of negative evaluation. Skills training as such may benefit the patient when sustained and intense pressures are placed upon the drinker and his worries interfere with rational replies. Maladaptive beliefs play a role here too ('It's a terrible thing if people think I'm unsociable').

In theory, assertiveness is a multi-layered process, but in practice it is not difficult to proceed with assertiveness therapy once the patient's mistaken beliefs are challenged and modified. Where there is boiling resentment just beneath a civil facade, or where people feel put upon but resist bringing the disagreement out into the open, assertion training will accomplish little until the patients come to understand that they can give up their deceptions and express disagreement without anger, depression and anxiety. Often the deceptions are excused on the grounds of altruism ('Because if I said I couldn't talk longer to my mother on the phone, or disagree with my wife over finances, it would hurt their feelings').Sissela Bok[16] writes trenchantly about such practices. 'All such deceptive practices claim benevolence [and] concern for the deceived . . . [While we must recognise the need] of not using truth as a weapon [it is true] that paternalistic lies . . . unlike so much deception, are felt to be without bias and are told in a disinterested wish [to be kind] . . . On closer examination, however, this objectivity and disinterest is often found to be spurious. The benevolent motives claimed by liars [a harsh but not inaccurate word for many instances of unassertiveness] are then seen to be mixed with many others, much less altruistic—the fear of confrontation which would accompany a more outspoken acknowledgement of the liar's feelings and intentions; the desire to avoid setting in motion great pressures to change, as when addiction is no longer concealed.' The costs? '[I]t questions . . . even the benefits that are thought to accrue to the liar. The effects of deception on the liars themselves—the need to shore up the lies, keeping them in good repair, the anxieties relating to positive discovery . . . are greatest in a close relationship where it is rare that one lie will suffice.'

The implementation begins with a search for the barriers that block assertive behaviour, especially fears. Another challenge must then be faced. Once the patient has a change of outlook he must accept that, for an initial period of time after he begins to behave in an assertive manner, he may be perceived as less friendly.[17] The therapist should take pains to state the obvious, that the other person's thoughts and evaluations are simply beyond the patient's control. When this crucial preliminary work and assessments have been done, assertiveness 'training' can then be started. The stages of skills acquisition are:

1. Cataloguing high risk situations.
2. Preparing new, assertive, responses.
3. Rehearsing these with the patient behaving as if it were a real situation. (The patient and the therapist should exchange roles from time to time, so that on occasions the patient plays the role of provocateur.)
4. Escalation from relatively easy to more demanding situations.

At all times it is important for the patient to communicate to the therapist estimates of the degree of strain or anxiety experienced in carrying out the role playing, even if done behaviourally to perfection. The smooth execution of an exercise in the clinic or elsewhere does not indicate that distress is necessarily absent. Working within the response inhibition model we put the greatest emphasis on the patient's feelings because these are the predictors of success or difficulties in assertion therapy.

Other techniques, contracting and counselling

The material in this chapter applies as much to controlled drinking goals as to abstinence. There are other kinds of advice and assistance which fit uniquely to controlled drinking goals. Controlled drinking is not a clinical method but an outcome. Here are certain useful guidelines which can help towards that end:

- Intoxication is associated with gulping rather than sipping drinks.
- Mixed drinks are preferable to straight spirits. (A nice point made by Sanchez-Craig is that when mixing drinks do not use carbonated mixers because they increase the absorption rate of alcohol.)
- Never drink on an empty stomach.

- Make a contract with a significant other before drinking (say, at a party) to space drinks (for example, one mixed drink or beer per hour). It is also helpful to use disclosure and contracting, with the drinker telling those he trusts about his plans and inviting them to lend a hand with reminders, collecting 'fines' for lapses, and keeping abreast of the patient's 'dry days', 'controlled days' and'lapses'.
- Make a commitment to alternate alcoholic with non alcoholic drinks or put double the amount of mixer in the drink.
- Avoid daily drinking.
- On drinking days keep to a limit of four standard drinks.
- Make the weekly limit 20 standard drinks for men (10 to 12 for women) and lower if necessary.

When the above goals, mutually agreed and not imposed, are met each day the drinker is advised to give himself a reward: points towards a trip or the purchase of a small item. He could have a little bank in the house where the money that would have been spent on excessive drinking can be deposited each day. Is this necessary? Virtue is said to be its own reward. Should not the fact that the patient is finished with ruinous drinking be enough in itself? Commonsense says 'Yes'; the data say 'Not necessarily'. Self-reward activities can be useful for a variety of possible reasons, perhaps because self-reward focusses the patient's attention each day on the work he has to do.

Other 'cognitive methods': family therapy

No theoretician or clinician, whatever his orientation to alcohol disorders, would expect the married problem drinker to be in harmony with his spouse and family. The close association between problem drinkers and family problems has led those in the family therapy movement to require that the drinker and every member of his family attend therapy. The reason for family treatments is that, in their view, alcoholism (or any psychological problem) is a family and not an individual disorder. In one sense this is true almost by definition. The effects of chronic heavy drinking and arguments about it will leave no one in that family untouched. The question is, how should the family be regarded: as 'patients' in a pathological family system, or should they take part as individuals who can learn to help the problem drinker by avoiding blame, giving up their own stereotypes, and acting cooperative with clinical goals?

Family therapy attempts to uncover the pathological beliefs and attitudes within the family system. Does it work? In a recent review Harwin[18] offered two conclusions about family therapy: a host of crucial issues are quite unresolved, and, on the whole, supposed benefits were not supported in evidence.

There are other forms of therapy which involve the family, though strictly speaking they are not 'family therapies'. In recent work with schizophrenics who were about to be discharged from hospital, it was shown that a psychoeducational approach designed to explain to the family the nature of the disorder and how to react assertively but calmly in difficult situations led to significantly fewer relapses than was the case in control subjects given the best individual therapy available. This therapy set as its goal the improvement of family/marital communication and problem solving. A 1985 marital therapy programme[19] run along these lines with problem drinkers and their spouses also produced encouraging results. Following the lead given by the schizophrenia researchers, where a good deal of excellent work has been done, members of the family should be taught how to express disagreement with the drinker without falling into the common traps and aversive habits of blame, destructive criticism and pessimism.

Cognitive therapy with the neurologically impaired

In 1979 Gorski and Miller described neurophysiological consequences of drinking which they labelled the 'post acute withdrawal syndrome' (PAW).[20] This notion was built on the assumption that the body's reaction to excessive drinking is a long-term homeostatic adjustment. When drinking is terminated withdrawal symptoms may appear, later abating over a period of a few days. Two weeks or so later the PAW is said to make its appearance, running a declining course over the next 12 weeks. Interestingly the same three month vulnerability period was uncovered by Hunt et al. in their review. Gorski and Miller hypothesise that PAW has an especially detrimental effect on the 'higher mental processes', including the ability to deal with abstractions, attention and memory. The PAW is also associated with an increase in response to stress. To date there are no standard batteries of tests for diagnosing a PAW reaction. The clinician is forced to rely on subjective reactions and overt signs which may include a collection of defensive reactions, avoidance of others, loss of planning abilities and perhaps severe depression. The serious implication for the use of cognitive therapy is memory loss of once-learned problem-solving strategies for high risk situations (Sanchez-Craig, personal communication). Signs of a PAW reaction would necessitate the use (and repetition) of simple, concrete cognitive therapies or perhaps the selection of other modes of therapy (see Chapter 9).

There is a general point to be taken from this discussion regardless of whether Gorski and Miller are precisely correct in the delineation of a PAW syndrome: therapies work best when they are matched to the conceptual level (CL) of the drinker. Those low in CL (say, as the result of permanent brain impairment) may do best with therapies that are highly structured and directive: 'Low CL patients appear to function best when rules are clear and . . . therapy style is clear, consistent, highly structured or directive'. The opposite is true of high CL patients. Thus cognitive-behaviour therapies would, following this advice, be appropriate for controlled drinkers-to-be or those in line for abstinence who are of at least average intelligence and without serious cognitive impairments. For all others, cognitive-behaviour therapies would appear to be premature during the first few weeks of therapy.

In closing, and to preserve a balance, it is worth repeating that the days of unimodal treatments of alcohol disorders should be behind us. Accordingly, advocates of cognitive-behaviour therapies must take care not to fall into the trap that for years has snared alcohol workers, which is getting locked into the belief that there is one ideal therapy (environmental, cognitive or biochemical) for problem drinking.

CHAPTER 11

Stress Management: Relaxation, Meditation and Hypnosis

It has long been accepted that alcoholics drink (a) to reduce dysphoria and (b) to obtain relief from tension, both physical and mental (i.e. worry). We have seen that there is no support for the first proposition. The available evidence, if anything, points in the opposite direction. *While* people are drinking to excess they suffer rising levels of distress and dysphoria. The *stated* goals, of enjoying improvements in mood while they are drinking, are goals which they fail to attain, every time.

The second assumption, the physical tension-reduction hypothesis, has been substantiated in a number of studies. The core proposition and the central claim of this hypothesis is that alcoholics suffer from high tension and that alcohol serves to reduce *physical* tension. Do problem drinkers experience higher level of tension than normal drinkers? When tension levels in problem drinkers are measured physiologically and compared with those in non-problem drinkers the findings are that 'alcoholics have a higher baseline of tension than do non-alcoholics'.[1] Second, when tension levels are monitored during alcohol consumption, reductions have been detected while at the same time adverse mood changes *increased*. In an important 1985 study Sandra Brown[2] searched for the alcohol-related expectancies in younger problem drinkers which would forecast the probability of a transition to excessive drinking. Of all the measures she used, 'The Tension Reduction Expectancy Scale' was identified as the best single predictor of a problematic drinking style. Although conclusions cannot be drawn from cross-sectional data, two hypotheses are suggested by these findings. First, individuals experiencing the reinforcing effects of greater degrees of tension reduction with alcohol consumption may be at risk for earlier problem drinking. The second, which is supported in clinical research, is that excessive drinkers will experience tension reduction from drinking[3] (whereas the effects on mood are in the opposite direction[4]). In one study, mentioned earlier, which tested shock aversion therapy in one group with that plus relaxation therapy in another, long-term abstinence rates were 23 per cent (not very different from the 'placebo' rates) and 46 per cent respectively. The absence of a control group rules out direct claims that relaxation as such was the sole reason for doubling the efficacy. Allowing for this methodological reserveration, it is safe to suppose that the relaxation did make a difference, but unqualified enthusiasm for relaxation must be tempered by the results of other investigations which found relaxation to be less promising for heavy drinkers who use alcohol for its (initial) euphoria-incentive effect.[5] Positive reports on the clinical value of relaxation training have come from investigations into the treatment of tension headaches, hypertension[6], sleep disturbances, and a host of other stress related disorders, as well as drinking disorders, including generalised anxiety, tension and worry.[7]

The literature on relaxation training suggests the following set of clarifications and guidelines for relaxation therapy:

1. The term 'relaxation training' has been used to describe a heterogenous pattern of practices which vary widely from one study to the next. (See King[8] for a useful discussion of this problem of terminological identity coupled with procedural diversity.)
2. Results are now available which help us to predict when and how to use relaxation procedures[9] and how such procedures may be misused:

   (a) Where there are no symptoms of physical tensions the technique will take up valuable clinical time to no effect.
   (b) Brief (less than two sessions) training is probably valueless.
   (c) Taped relaxation procedures in this, as in all areas of therapy, are inferior to live training.
   (d) Relaxation, properly taught, is most effective when it can be used in or before interpersonal stress situations in order to enhance a sense of perceived control in that situation.
   (e) Hence drinkers should be taught to apply relaxation therapy *in their daily activities* and not just during practice sessions.

Two more important points deserve mention. First, many alcoholics are demonstrably poor at discriminating levels and kinds of tension. Accordingly one of the aims of relaxation therapy should be to promote the awareness of excessive tension in everyday stress situations as well as its management. Second, it is now recognised that while mental tensions and worries are characteristic of some problem drinkers, physical tensions are more of a difficulty for others. The clinician should aim to match the client to the appropriate technique.

One of these, biofeedback makes use of sensitive measuring devices to record subtle and ongoing activities in a particular part of the body. The technique involves giving the patient information about moment-to-moment changes in the operation of a particular organ or system. A light or buzzer or some other cue is used to indicate to the patient that small but important progress towards the goal of better functioning is underway. With instantaneous feedback and extensive training individuals have been taught to alter various activities going on within their own bodies. This has been of great theoretical and experimental interest. Cardiovascular, autonomic and central nervous system activities once believed to be involuntary can be brought under 'voluntary' control and pathological or excessive reactions corrected.

These demonstrations notwithstanding, there are serious doubts about the applicability of biofeedback relaxation training to alcoholism. Biofeedback requires complex, sophisticated electronic equipment (the cheaper 'do-it-yourself-at-home' devices are worthless) under the direction of a practitioner with expert training. Most clinicians do not have the background or the technology to offer effective biofeedback training. Then there is the question of 'generalisability'. While people can perform in the laboratory, under the guidance of the biofeedback expert, it remains to be established that the patient can 'turn on' the same effects without the help of the right equipment and the presence of the specialist. Looking into this matter, Lehrer[10] finished a review of the clinical biofeedback work with a forceful statement of these doubts: 'The results strongly indicate that biofeedback is not a useful treatment component for the reduction of anxiety or physiological arousal when compared with live, carefully administered relaxation instructions; and it is certainly not a substitute for the latter.'

In the following sections we describe two relaxation techniques in some detail: Jacobson's deep muscle relaxation procedure and non-cult meditation. These are two of the best and easiest techniques to teach as *methods for coping* with physical and mental tensions respectively. Meditation therapy has another important aim in addition which is the control of 'worry' which distinguishes it from relaxation therapies directed at tension problems alone.

Rationale

In Chapter 10 emphasis was given to the crucial role a coherent and persuasive rationale plays in raising levels of compliance. For the clinician to know that technique X or Y has solid support in evidence is only half the story; the other half is transmitting this to the patient, clearly and in nontechnical language. If properly done, this can have a motivating as well as an educational effect. The rationale plus the diary record of homework exercises can significantly increase compliance rates and, thereby, therapeutic results.

The following is the justification to be given to the patient before embarking on relaxation training. For the most part, patients accept the value of relaxation as a general aim. But even if they take this as self-evident, the significance of the muscle relaxation procedures may not be apparent if the mechanisms are not outlined. Patients often wonder how their needs will be served by a relaxation technique which begins with an *increase* in muscle tension. While they may appreciate the desirability of relaxation, they may well be unaware of the psychological costs of chronic tension. It is therefore essential that an introduction to progressive relaxation should incorporate clarifying remarks on both these aspects. The therapist should use an approach of this sort:

> 'We all appreciate that relaxation is probably a good thing, but most of us may not realise that what is happening with our muscles can make the difference between being "up-tight" and being relaxed. The first thing to remember is that when we contract our muscles [this can be demonstrated by the therapist tensing his hands and shoulders], we are doing *work*. This means that energy is being expended, lost. Note that whether or not this work achieves a useful purpose is beside the point. Take the example of two men, Mr Andrews and Mr Brown. Mr

Andrews 'spends' a certain amount of energy painting his house. Mr Brown expends exactly the same amount of time and energy sitting tense at work all day. As far as Mr Andrews is concerned, the muscle contractions which he used when painting his house were productive; for Mr Brown, sitting tense at his desk, the work was wasted. But the decline in energy levels was the same in both cases. As another example, we have Mr Collins and Mr Drew, who work side-by-side at the same job. Mr Collins' levels of muscle tension are exactly what he needs to get the job done properly. Mr Drew is twice as tense. One could say that Mr Drew therefore works a 16-hour day, or a 10-day week. But, of course, the company is not going to pay him twice as much or double his vacation period. Actually, in this example, Mr Drew would not only be more up-tight than his work-mate but his job efficiency would probably suffer as well. So the first reason to learn to control muscle tension, all over the body, is to free oneself from fatigue. As you know from your own experience, the more worn out you are, the more easily you can become emotionally upset.

There is a second reason for learning and practicing the skills of muscle relaxation. Anxiety, frustration and other unpleasant moods feed on muscle tension. I don't mean to say that being tense is the same thing as being frustrated, anxious or emotionally distressed. I can make my right hand and arm very tense [demonstrate] but I'm no more upset now than I was 10 seconds ago. However, had I been, say, anxious before I did that, for whatever reason, then muscle tension could have added to it, especially if I had kept it up for a long time, as people often do. One way it does this is by increasing the physical changes which are at work in depression, anger and anxiety. To give one example, when we tense our muscles, we can increase the speed and intensity of cardiovascular activity. People often report that when they are anxious they are aware of their heart pounding. Using muscle relaxation exercises during times of anxiety can help to slow down these unpleasant reactions and thus help to reduce anxiety.

Thirdly, in addition, excessive muscle tension can also be highly distracting, creating 'inner' noise which interferes with our performance of everyday activities.

Turning now to the remedy, there is no one method alone by

which relaxation can be achieved. There are a number that are widely used. These can be divided into two types—those which emphasise techniques of producing 'mental calm', such as meditation, where it is expected that physical relaxation will automatically follow, and others which begin with physical relaxation training in the hope that mental calm will accompany it. Our practice is to teach both, each of which will help the other. The one we're going to start with is called progressive muscle (or sometimes 'deep muscle') relaxation and it is widely used for eliminating physical tension.

The exercises are not difficult, involving only a sequence of tensing and relaxing movements in various parts of the body. Though it may seem odd that we should begin with tensing the muscles, given that this is all about relaxation, the reason is that when we are under stress, muscle tension can be fairly high and persist without our being aware of it. By first making the muscles tense, you can learn how to develop a kind of automatic "tension detector".'

Patient estimates of muscle tension: quantitative or qualitative?
All the relaxation methods with which we are familiar call upon the patient to make distinctions between higher and lower levels of tension, but the requests are communicated and assessed in qualitative terms ('I was fairly tense yesterday when I was called upon to say a few words at the wedding' or, 'make your right hand very tense', etc.). The imprecision of this practice can be overcome by using the TT (tension thermometer). Thus we say to the patient:

'In our practice I'll be asking you to "turn on" different amounts of tension in various muscle groups, or I may ask you *how* tense you are at a given time, or to rate how much tension you felt at some other time [in the bar, arriving home after a frustrating day, or whatever the patient's stress situation]. Phrases like 'a lot' or 'a little' or 'terribly high' may not mean the same to you as they do to me, and what I mean by them may not be clear to you. To get around this problem we can use an imaginary 100 point measuring scale. At the bottom is zero, which means no tension in *that part of the body* [be sure that the patient realises that here specific and not global ratings are requested] and "100" means as much tension as you could make in that part. I'll show you what I mean. Look at my right hand. See how relaxed it is? I'd give it a number somewhere between "0" and "10". Now [therapist makes a loose fist] it's not much higher—I'd say about "10" to "15" on the tension scale [by modelling the use of a quick estimate of tension levels, the therapist can forestall worries in the patient that he must be *exactly* precise in the numbers he uses]. I'll increase it to about "30". See the difference? And now up to "50" . . . now its at "90" to "100" [fist and arm shaking with the effort].'

Tension changes: gradual or abrupt?

All the manuals we have consulted agree on the *timing* of tension release—to be done during exhalation—but not on the amount to be relaxed. It is known that a slight, unconditioned, reflexive, easing of tension occurs when we exhale and, conversely, a slight tendency to increase muscle tension as we inhale. By pairing relaxation with the outflow of breath, we can capitalise on this natural contingency. But how much tension is to be let out during exhalation? In some systems the patient is asked to release a barely perceptible amount with each breath, while others request the patient to 'let it all go at once'.[11] Despite the popularity of both methods, there has been little debate over the advisability of one over the other. We find the general indifference to the question puzzling, for patients usually report a strong preference for the 'all-at-once' release. Quite apart from the greater satisfaction, there are other reasons for the abrupt-decrease method. Chronically tense individuals typically show a poor awareness of tension levels and a corresponding difficulty in detecting small changes in these. Beginning with the general principle that discrimination learning will always proceed most rapidly when training begins with large differences before the subject is called upon to discriminate more subtle differences,[12] it makes sense for tension-release instructions to emphasise the quick, abrupt mode of release in the target areas. In discussing the merits of the two, Malmo[13] referred to a number of EMG reports of muscle tension (EMG standing for electromyograph, a procedure for measuring changes in the activity of specific muscles). He wrote that 'the rate of terminal fall also seems of psychological significance. A *prompt, large* drop generally coincides with successful completion of a task, giving the person a "feeling of closure". A much slower fall in muscle tension, on the other hand, is usually associated with something not quite complete or not fully satisfying about the performance' (emphasis added).

This is not to say that the therapist should always ask the patient to generate and sustain maximal (i.e. '100') level so as to get the greatest possible drop on the release phase. Indeed, we can see two reasons not to ask for the maximum possible amount of tension at the beginning of each subroutine. First, achieving and holding '100' levels is very fatiguing, and some patients feel the disturbing after-effects of such efforts well after the signal to 'return to zero.' Second, even chronically tense patients rarely experience maximal tension in their everyday lives. The problem is not that they become *that* tense, but that they get up to and stay at intermediate levels for long periods of time.[14] Thus we advise spending most of the training time working within the '40' to '70' range, with the aim of maximising transfer and increasing the 'ecological validity' of progressive muscle relaxation therapy.

Duration of cycles and areas targeted

There are a number of related questions to consider under this heading. The first is the duration of a given tension-release cycle. The ideal length is not known, but most manuals that offer a recommendation on this point advise 25 seconds or less. We have found it helpful for the patient to hold the requested level in the nominated muscle group for two breathing cycles (i.e., between 15 and 20 seconds). Much shorter durations than that do not permit the patients to 'tune into' and study the tension-related sensations, and ones longer than that can be tiring and unpleasant.

Second, we can ask about the number of repetitions in any given target muscle group. Once again there is no good data base on which to form a decision. Our advice is that it is probably desirable to have more than one trial with a particular muscle group, but just how many more will depend on the patient's ability to get down to and stay within the '0' to '10' range following release. Also important is the site where the individual experiences the worst tension in stress situations. Some people may be predominantly face responders, others back or arm responders, and so on. The greatest attention and the most practice should be given to particular trouble spots. If the therapist elects to do all of the major voluntary muscles (a standard sequence is: hands, biceps and triceps, shoulders, neck, forehead, eyes, lips, tongue [pressed into the roof of the mouth], back, midsection, thighs, calves, feet and toes; see below for detailed instructions to the patient), extra practice should be schedules for the individual's problem areas (which are often to be found in the hands, face, lips, forehead, eyes, arms, and neck and shoulders).

Finally, the duration of training overall is an issue. Our experience, which is in line with the available research,[15] indicates that at least two 40 minute sessions will be required. How many more than that will depend on the extent of the problem and the goals in therapy.

Problems

Although patients are instructed to isolate the requested tension to the target areas, the 'migration' of tension to other muscles is to be expected. Patients will need many reminders, *during training*, to keep the tension localised. One way to inhibit this spread is to give repeated emphasis to the importance of maintaining the integrity of the breathing rhythm. Tense patients almost always either stop breathing altogether or breathe too deeply and strenuously during the tension induction phase.

Certain muscle groups appear to be more prone to cramping (for example, the shoulder-neck area when hunched, the underside of the thighs, and the arches of the feet when the toes are tensed). Care must be taken in these areas to keep the tension below '70' in individuals who show any tendency to experience muscle spasms and cramps.

Sample exercise

The one sketched out below is the 'hand exercise,' but the same delivery is used for all the other muscle groups. The first set of instructions in any area will always be more lengthy than they will need to be on repetitions of the cycle.

> 'Now that you have a nice easy breathing rhythm be sure that you don't let the tension which you will be producing interfere with your breathing. I'd like you to continue as though your breathing didn't "know" anything about the tensing or relaxing. Good. All right, in a minute or so I'm going to ask you to make your right hand into a fist, fingers flat against your

palms so that your fingernails don't dig into them and then raise the tension to "70" [or whatever level] until I signal to let release the tension. One more thing: as I said earlier, make certain that you get up to the "70" level before you finish inhaling the breath on which I ask you to begin. By the time you get to the 'top' of that breath, so to speak, you should be at "70". After two cycles of in and out breathing I'll ask you to let all that tension go *as you are breathing out*. And it should all be gone before you complete the outbreath on which I ask you to release the tension. In other words before you get to the 'bottom' of that breath, and certainly before you begin the next breath in, the tension level in your hand should be as close to zero as you can let it be.

OK, let's start. The next breath *after* this one, make your right hand into a fist and go up the tension scale until you get to "70" or thereabouts . . . good [if the patient stops breathing or starts breathing too deeply remind him to return to steady breathing]. Don't let the tension start anywhere else . . . now study the sensations you feel in your hand and up to your forearm, pay attention to them . . . good . . . next breath out, let it *all* go . . . that's it . . . notice the difference between the tension you felt a few seconds ago and what you are presently experiencing in your right hand . . . if you notice any "leftover" tension just let it slip away the next time you exhale.' (The therapist can also ask the patient to notice the quiet and the calm he feels, and 'how much nicer it is' in the absence of high tension levels.)

Additions and variations

After going through the complete cycle (hands, arms, etc.) the therapist can have the patient superimpose the word 'tense' whenever muscle tension is increased (i.e., as he breaths in) and the word 'relax' with tension release (on exhalation). This is known as *cue-controlled relaxation.*[16] This gives the patient cognitive control over muscle tension and can deepen his awareness of what is going on in his body. (After constant practice with the use of these cues, patients tell us things like: 'It was surprising the other day when I was held up in a traffic jam; I started to get pretty wound up and then I "heard" the word "tense" in my head and it reminded me to relax.')

When patients are accomplished in the use of progressive relaxation in the clinic and during daily home practice (i.e., in optimal conditions), we ask them to do daily, short (less than 3 minutes) exercises in the face of self-imposed stressors (for example, making the shower colder; turning on the radio so that the station selection device gets two programmes at once, or static). This is a kind of 'stress inoculation'[17] which can, in addition, promote generalisation from the safety and security of the practice situation to the rigors of their real-life encounters with tension and stress.

Finally, a reminder. With progressive relaxation, as with all of the other techniques mentioned in this book, daily home practice and the associated record keeping must be built into the programme and reviewed at each clinical meeting.

The effects of meditation therapy

The use of non-cult, or secular, meditation is of recent origin in clinical practice. The main premise of progressive relaxation is that physical tension can produce psychological problems. Meditation theory is predicated on the opposite—but not rival—premise that 'mental calm' can have a positive influence on the physical reactions going on throughout the body. When meditation was first introduced proponents went further and claimed that it produced greater changes than any other (non-meditation) relaxation method and that it led to a set of alterations which were 'unique' and unattainable by any other means. Investigators have since come to different conclusions. Meditation practice is as good as, but not better than, progressive relaxation in eliciting lowered arousal and the counter anxiety/stress responses which are of great interest to the clinician working with alcoholic patients.[18]

While there are some differences—meditation, for example, may be superior to progressive relaxation in combating intrusive, worrying thoughts—both seem to produce a common, integrated 'relaxation response'. Benson[19] coined this term to describe the coordinated collection of changes which make a clear contrast with the 'flight fight' pattern evoked in situations of worry, anxiety, panic and fear. Lehrer et al.[20] favour meditation, despite the fact that their extensive study showed it to be roughly equivalent in effectiveness to relaxation (or even slightly less so) because 'meditation appears to be more motivational for most people . . . [they] appeared to enjoy meditation more. They practised it [significantly] more and reported being more involved in the technique.' This has been the finding in the University of New South Wales Psychology Clinic. The same was found by Glueck and Stroebel.[21] They devised an experiment which they hoped would give information about the comparative value of relaxation, biofeedback and meditation. To their surprise they were not able to complete the experiment. Virtually all of the (psychiatric) patients in the biofeedback and relaxation groups complained that they found the daily practice sessions extremely tedious and the majority dropped out of the experiment. Those in the meditation group not only continued with their practices but also reported that they enjoyed it and recommended it to their friends.

To conclude, meditation can help to combat the otherwise powerful tendencies to excessive worry and tension which burden the alcoholic. Other techniques or just the simple recommendation to sit and listen to pleasant music can also effect positive changes[22]. But the biofeedback machine or the pleasant music may not be available when needed. Meditation is our first preference because it is 'portable'. It can be used at any time, is unobtrusive when used in public, and reduces the patient's dependence on external supports.

Meditation therapy: an introduction

Meditation, once regarded as exotic and esoteric, has recently become known to the non-specialist practitioner and the layman. In fact it is being popularised by enthusiastic teachers to the extent that there is a risk that it will be oversold as a panacea for all ailments. Too often those associated with one variety of meditation are at pains to distinguish their 'brand' from what they consider to be inferior rivals. However, until there is evidence to indicate the superiority of one variety, the claims for any one as *the* technique of meditation must be rejected. Indeed there is reason to wonder if there are really substantial differences between the various techniques beyond the obvious surface details. Some forms of meditation require the student to sit in the quiet contemplation of certain objects or pictures. Others are built around unusual breathing rhythms. Then there are teachers of meditation who give their students special phrases (mantras) to repeat.

To the newcomer meditation would seem to comprise a bewildering variety of techniques. On closer examination, though, it is possible to discern commonalities. Most forms contain the following three recommendations. First, meditation should take place somewhere free from excessive noise and distractions. Second, the meditator should adopt a comfortable position, either seated or lying down, in which he should be able to relax, while at the same time not be in danger of falling asleep. Third, the meditator should be given certain behavioural or mental routines which are to be repeated for the duration of the meditation practice. These can be movements, or mental exercises which involve the repetition of a particular word or phrase. While the meditator is engaged in these routines he is warned against 'trying' of any sort, whether to relax or to solve problems. Eugen Herrigel[23] beautifully described the preferred attitude of the meditator as that of a person engaged in the 'artless art' or the 'effortless effort'.

When meditation is reduced to these few guidelines it appears to be a very simple technique. In one sense it is: meditation benefits from and encourages an attitude of unforced simplicity. In another sense it is not: acquiring proficiency at meditation takes understanding, time and training.

Teaching meditation therapy

When the topic of meditation is introduced in therapy, patients either embrace the idea immediately or pull back with reservations. The hesitant ones usually change their attitude when they find out what meditation has accomplished for others. The eager ones will have heard stories, often exaggerated, of the 'wonders of meditation'. Securing an in-principle acceptance of meditation for purposes of stress management is never a difficult task: it is when discussion turns to the question of detail and technique that problems crop up. Once the basics of meditation are outlined patients invariably react with disbelief: 'Is that all there is to it?' The disparity between the simple procedures of meditation and the far-reaching changes which it sets in train seems to violate the conventional wisdom that only complex methods can produce complex results.

The therapist can respond to the patient's doubts by choosing to overlook them and simply press on with the techniques of meditation therapy. Patients will generally go along for a while with the directions of an authoritarian therapist and a few may even carry on for long enough to acquire the skills and to reap the benefits. However most will give up the programme, using excuses such as 'I meant to do the practice but the week was so busy I couldn't find the time'. A better approach is to give the patient a reasonably good grasp of how meditation works and how best to use it, and to acquaint him with the problems which he may encounter along the way *before the practice itself is begun.* Having been introduced to meditation in this way the informed patient will persist with it for longer, and will get much more out of it, than the patient who is simply told what to do.

The control of breathing

There are two related findings which reveal close connections between the way we breathe and feelings of tension. Very fast breathing, hyperventilation, can trigger a number of stress reactions including disturbing 'tingling' feelings in the hands and arms, mental confusion and dizziness. If left unchecked, hyperventilation can lead to panicky feelings. The reverse is true of slow breathing: it facilitates relaxation and a sense of calmness and control. Regular, steady breathing is emphasised in meditation training, making the patient aware of patterns of respiration and their importance. It can take some while, much practice, and many reminders before the correct control of breathing in challenging situations becomes as automatic as overbreathing once had been.

The control of worry by the training of attention

Meditation is an indirect means of combating negative, worrisome thinking. ('Worry' as we are using it here refers to anxious apprehension and other maladaptive, self-defeating thoughts which may be associated with affective reactions of anger, depression or frustration.) This is accomplished by giving the patient more control over the direction of his attention. Because we attach great significance to the attentional-control function of meditation we have gone to some lengths in the remainder of this section to amplify these points. In particular, our aim in the following paragraphs is, first, to show the connection between thoughts and feelings and then to highlight the even more important relationship between attention and thought. The ultimate objective is to indicate how meditation can be taught, and used, as an attentional control technique (and hence of the thought-feeling sequence).

In order to illustrate the important relationship between attention and thought, let us begin with a description of a standard experimental arrangement designed to explore the links between thought and emotion. A person with a well-established distress reaction to certain situations (for example, being criticised) is asked to sit on a comfortable recliner chair in a quiet room. Once the equipment to measure his reactions is in place, he is told to think about a pleasant scene. After continuing with this for a few moments a number of measurable changes will be recorded: these will include a slowing of respiration, a decline in heart rate and a number of other obvious and subtle changes consistent with his calm 'state of mind'. He is then asked to summon up a mental picture of a scene filled with his personal stressors. After this he is asked to fill his thoughts with the kind of self-talk which would usually occupy his mind when he is in the real stress situation, such as 'Oh, this is awful. I'm getting angry (upset, etc.). I could use a drink!' Although no stress stimulus is physically present the recording instrument will show marked reversals as the physical signs of relaxation are replaced by stress reactions, perhaps less pronounced but of the same kind as those which would appear in the presence of the stress stimulus itself.

What do such changes demonstrate? They show that we have the ability to create stress reactions, or the reverse, by changing our patterns of thought. Our person 'moved' from deep relaxation to pronounced stress without leaving the chair or opening his eyes. (Emotions other than anxiety have also been produced in this way: depressed moods have been created in subjects instructed to think of self-statements of failure and deprecation.[24] In addition to making us aware of the intimate relationship between thought and feeling they also illustrate another and perhaps less obvious point: we can choose, to some extent, the stimuli to which we will react by giving our attention to them. At any instant we can 'select' the inner or outer stimuli in which we will become absorbed. The activities, things or memories thus selected exert a powerful influence on the emotional tone of our feelings for as long as we remain absorbed in them. The absorption, or to use the word we prefer, the attention to the things going on around and within us, is the key element in the worry process. As I write this passage I could stop for a moment and turn my attention to an encounter with an unfriendly colleague which is scheduled for tomorrow afternoon. If my thoughts are filled with anticipation of an unpleasant interaction then my mood will mirror the content of these thoughts. Alternatively, I could disengage my attention from anticipation of this meeting, though perhaps not immediately, and elect instead to turn it back to, say, some pleasant interlude from the past. There are still other options open to me. Instead of giving 'centre stage' to thoughts of the past or the future I could turn away from my desk and look out of the window at the street scene outside, or I could scan and select for attention any of the large number of things in my immediate environment. Whether I 'fill up my mind' by looking forward or backward in time, or within or around me, will hinge on how I deploy my attention. Attention is the psychological 'filter' of the mind.

What does all of this say about 'worry'? We began with illustrations of the thought-feeling sequence of worry. With the inclusion of 'attention' we have arrived at a more complex sequence. It must now read: worry is the (a) selection of/attention to, and thus production of (b) negative thoughts of apprehension and failure, which (c) are correlated with the emotional reactions/physical changes which are a reflection of these thoughts.

If we find a person whose attention is drawn to patterns of thinking that have an intrusive, 'attention' capturing quality about them, we call that person a 'worrier'. Alcoholics are chronic worriers. People do not simply react to challenges as they arise nor do they merely register attacks of anger, anxiety or depression when an active dispute comes to pass. They tend to worry about things that might happen. Alcoholics may worry when they try to cope with the anticipated presence of drink, or anticipated arguments and the problem drinking that has so often followed. The inability of the drinker to control his attention can exact a terrible toll. The drinker is, in a sense, rehearsing failure or reminding himself of past slips. The effects of this activity feed forward so that when he finds himself embroiled in high-risk situations his attention is pulled toward images of failing and drinking. He is likely to combine these with self-talk that is ill-advised in the extreme, ensuring that his worst anticipations will come true.

We have mentioned the two obvious costs of worry: immediate stress and the long-term erosion of confidence. We have not yet mentioned the third cost: the loss of enjoyment in everyday activities. When we lose (attentional) contact with the activities of the present and, inadvertently, focus our attention on intrusive and irrelevant thoughts, we pay a price. An example should make this clear. Suppose that while I am at a restaurant getting ready to eat a meal I become preoccupied with the recall of a recent frustrating encounter with a difficult patient. How would this affect the 'enjoyability quotient' of the meal? The answer is that it would all depend on how much attention I paid to the food and how much to the competing activity (for example, the recall of yesterday's disappointments). If we measure the attention given to something (meal, recall, anticipation, the person across the room) on a scale of '0' ('completely oblivious') to '100' ('fully engrossed'), then if my attention is equally divided between the memory and the meal (an attention rating to the meal of '50') my enjoyment of it would be reduced by a corresonding amount. By comparison, if I were completely caught up in this 'excursion' away from the meal (i.e., giving the excursion an attention rating of '100') then my enjoyment of the meal would be absolutely nil. The result? The potentially pleasurable activity of eating the meal would be reduced to the mechanical act of consumption.

Can anything be done about worry? Rephrased to fit in with our analysis of the stress sequence, the question becomes: can anything be done to give the patient control of the direction of his attention? The importance of attention as the key to 'the portals of the mind' (nowadays psychologists would use the expression 'the control of cognition') was a central theme in the writings of the eminent nineteenth century philosopher-doctor-psychologist William James. His often-quoted words on the subject of attention refer to the fact that our emotional reactions, indeed the very quality of our lives, are powerfully affected by the direction of our attention: 'Each of us literally chooses, by his ways of attending to things, what sort of universe he shall appear to himself to inhabit'.[25] This gives due recognition to the role of attention but it does not tell us if we can learn to discipline the mind and thus influence our emotional lives by the control of attention. Can we, as Bligh put it in 1910 'be the gardeners of our inclinations. . . . Can we as richly and advantageously cultivate the germs of anger, pity, inquisitiveness, vanity [and anxiety/worry] as we train a beautiful fruit along the wall?' Today we have evidence that people can learn to control their attentional processes. 'A growing body of data indicates that humans can acquire some degree of control . . . [and] one of the oldest techniques for achieving such self regulation is meditation.[26]

Questions about meditation

When this section on meditation, attention and the control of worry was in preparation we sought out the views and reactions of a number of therapists and clinical research scientists. Although the overall response was positive, once we presented our rationale in detail, certain requests for amplification and comment came up again and again in discussions. As 'worry' is a neglected topic, we felt it may be useful to list these recurring questions and our clarifications. Cognitive therapy is a term which refers to a set of techniques for helping patients examine their negative thought patterns. The search is for fallacious assumptions contained within their inner talk and chains of ideas and imagery. Using logic and reason, patients are taught to attack the mistaken assumptions underlying faulty thinking about themselves, others, and their problems. Cognitive therapy is therefore very different from training for the control of attention. In meditation ('attentional therapy' might be another name for it) the person practices how to 'step back' from intrusive thoughts that lead him on by degrees to the first drink or the first drink too many. The difference between cognitive therapy and meditation turns on the contrasting approaches toward stress provoking thoughts. In meditation they are not to be probed, analysed or disputed, as in cognitive therapy. Instead, the patient is taught how to gently dismiss unprofitable thinking by withdrawing from it the focus of attention. Both have a role to play. We believe that they are complementary to one another.

You have said that meditation therapy also teaches patients to become tuned into and to practise control over breathing. That seems a reasonable objective. But isn't this other business of 'avoiding the pitfalls of negative thinking by denying it our atten-

tion', simply a matter of ignoring instead of facing the problem—sweeping it under the carpet, so to speak?
We agree that 'facing the problem' is an unavoidable part of treatment. Cognitive therapy, relapse therapy and general counselling are all predicated upon the belief that 'facing the problem' is the best way to conquer challenges. Indeed these techniques deliberately involve the patient in thinking about his problems. The patient is provided with imaginal or vicarious exposure to them in the discussion, planning, and evaluation stage. For example in relapse therapy, patients are asked to visualise themselves entering high-risk situations and practicing coping techniques where in the past drinking has got out of control. Do the positive findings from the use of these techniques contradict our position on the value of attentional control? We do not think so. The fact is that in meditation, as in cognitive therapy, care is taken to help the patient keep clear of chronic immersion in self-defeating, unrealistic, fright- and failure-oriented thinking and being overwhelmed by excessively stressful feelings.

What is the difference between attention training and thought stopping techniques?
The family of techniques known by the term 'thought stopping' also recognises that there is a close interplay between thought and feeling. Where they differ from meditation therapy for attention training is that they require a direct 'attack' on negative thoughts or images, for example, by first deliberately inducing the patient to produce the offending cognition and then having him shout aloud or say to himself: 'STOP'—perhaps augmenting the impact by visualising a traffic stop sign. It is proposed that the chain of upsetting negative thoughts can be inhibited or overridden by these dramatic interventions.

This is quite different from the counselling given to the patient trained in meditation: 'When you stray "off course", when thoughts of failure come to mind, don't struggle against them. Let the thoughts come and go as they please; your job is to ensure that you do not give them the full focus of your attention. How? You can avoid being trapped in a web of destructive thoughts and feelings by "stepping back" from them and reinvolving your attention in the exercise routine (if it happens during the daily practice periods) or in your everyday life on ongoing events.' In recommending to the patient that he adopt an attitude of tolerant indifference to and distance from 'catastrophising' thoughts he is, in effect, being told: 'Look, these thoughts should be given the significance they deserve, which is no great significance at all'.

In our laboratory my colleagues and I tested attentional control versus thought stopping techniques (both with eyes closed) in different groups of volunteers given neutral or upsetting thoughts as targets. The object of the exercise was to see in which of the two conditions the 'prohibited' thoughts intruded more often. (The volunteers were to raise their fingers whenever this happened.) The subjects given thought stopping directions and training reported more than three times as many intrusions as the meditation subjects.

We will stay on this point a little longer because patients often misconstrue the purpose of meditation training in this regard. To drive home the point we might say 'O.K., if you think you can "do battle" with intrusive thoughts and make your mind a "clean slate", try this. For the next 20 seconds do not think of the word "camel" and do not get a mental image of one, either.' Patients discover that they can do nothing of the kind. We go on 'Well, that wasn't a great success; perhaps it will be easier with the word "newspaper". Same as before—do not think of it for the next 20 seconds.' Once again the patient fails. We finish with 'Let's have one more trial: Oklahoma—do not think of the state of Oklahoma.' When the patient records yet another 'failure' we ask 'By the way, what happened with "camel"? It has gone, hasn't it?' We concluded by pointing out 'You stopped thinking about "camel" the instant you stopped trying to stop—when you turned your attention away from it.'

When you quote William James' remarks about each of us 'choosing' the world we inhabit, and, by extension, our emotional responses to it, and when you talk about the 'selection' of thoughts, are you saying that the patient has complete discretion as to the internal or external things in which he shall become 'involved'?

Very much to the contrary. Before patients learn about the interconnections between attention, thought and feeling, they cause themselves untold extra distress through prolonged involvement with failure imagery, negative self-talk and misinterpretations of ordinary events. Once this realisation is acquired it is essential for patients to accept the need for consistent practice before they can transform it into a reliable skill. On the way to this objective we make it clear that at the first attempt to exercise this 'choice' they will become painfully aware of how much of a challenge it is to gain control over the 'unruly' attention and the 'unquiet' mind.

You seem to be saying that all emotional upheavals begin with the attention-thought sequence which concludes in the negative feelings. Are you ignoring sudden physiological upheavals, aversive feelings like sudden 'spontaneous' depressions and anxiety, a large proportion of which are described by patients as 'out of the blue' and strongly physical, reactions of fear? In the same vein are nonconscious thought processes excluded from your system?
Our answer is 'No' to both questions. As so many patients discover, the onset of some disruptive physical changes can be hastened by chronic negative thinking. Other reactions, though, do indeed seem to come *before* and not after 'negative thinking'. Nonetheless, a vicious cycle can be established very quickly if the patient loses control over his attention and is trapped in anticipations of failure and relapse.

As regards the existence of nonconscious mental activities, they once were, but are no longer, denied. The real issue is whether the cognitive activities which go on out of awareness are sufficient by themselves to trigger sustained and strong emotional reactions. To that we can only answer: possibly they are but probably they are not. If research data come to hand which indicate that nonconscious mental activity can directly evoke the changes which make up physical states of emotion, our attention and interpretations will still contribute to the persistence of aversive feelings that come to our awareness. So, whichever position is the correct one we must still pay attention to 'attention'.

Techniques of meditation

Preparation

For meditation to be successful it is first necessary for there to be a special place where the exercise is to be done. Ideally, it should be done in that same place twice a day for about 20 minutes each time. The meditation room should be quiet, dimly lit, and located away from household activities. If other people are in the house at meditation times they should be requested to stay away from the area while the patient is practising and to answer the telephone or the doorbell so that the meditation period is not beset by interruptions. Preparation should also include the arrangement of a post-meditation period of a few minutes of free time after the conclusion of the meditation itself. If such an allowance is not made, anticipation of whatever tasks the person must begin immediately afterwards will intrude and pose a significant obstacle to the centering or control of attention—the main objective of meditation.

When to meditate

There is no conclusive evidence to prove that meditation should be undertaken at certain times and not others but patients seem to find that once at lunchtime, before eating, and once again in the early evening are generally the best times. Most find that it is best not to meditate just after a big meal (although no one has yet produced hard evidence to confirm this belief). It is inadvisable to undertake the second of the two meditation periods late in the evening or at a time when sleepy or fatigued. Being in a softly lit and quiet room with the eyes closed and the body in a comfortable posture can make sleep irresistible and, for that reason, meditation impossible.

Posture and meditation

Some schools of meditation insist that the student hold a particular posture for the duration of the practise, such as the 'lotus position'. No evidence has come to light on the value of one posture over another and the experimental literature shows no link between posture in meditation and clinical outcomes. We suggest only that the patient be comfortable and relaxed while meditating. This is more easily achieved if the patient loosens tight clothing, removes spectacles and keeps legs uncrossed. It is probably better if meditation is done in a chair instead of on a bed. Even if fatigue is low and it is not late, the association between a prone position in bed and sleep may be too strong for some. In effect then, there is also a recommendation for the ideal posture here: the patient should meditate in a place and position which will allow for relaxation without promoting sleep.

Breathing and meditation
In the literature on meditation there are many instructions but few facts about the best style of breathing. Nevertheless there is widespread agreement that diaphragmatic breathing is preferable to high, shallow breathing. Some teachers of meditation also counsel the deliberate pacing of breathing according to some predetermined rhythm. We have tried this but have now abandoned it in favour of the simpler instructions: 'Breathe easily and without effort. You don't need to breathe very deeply and certainly not quickly.' We add: 'Let your breathing settle, gradually, into a nice steady rhythm. Breathe through your nose, silently, quietly and easily.' It is probably inadvisable to stress the need for patients deliberately to regulate the rate of breathing for, if such advice is given, the ideal in meditation of an easy, non-striving attitude (the 'effortless effort') will be difficult to maintain.

Mental activities in meditation
Finally, there is the most important part of meditation—the mental activities in which the patient is to engage for the 20 minute period. The guiding instruction is for the patient to make use of an attentional 'anchor'. This can take the form of a word, phrase and/or movement which is to be repeated over and over for the whole of the period. The objective is for the patient to practise organising his attention and awareness around the 'here and now' activitity which he has been given. By using the mental routines of meditation the patient can learn the skills (and appreciate the importance) of gently resisting the capture of his attention by intrusive thoughts concerned with his anxieties, or for that matter, with any irrelevant material. The particular word, phrase or routine used does not possess any intrinsic importance. The point is for the patient to become proficient at controlling the attention towards chosen external and mental events.

In practice, at the outset at least, this will be no easy matter, as he will soon discover. Without exception, people complain that they 'automatically' move away from the centering activity and onto something else. When pulled away from the mental routine of meditation the repetitive activity provides the 'home base' to return to after each 'excursion'. Patients find that every time they practise disengaging from passing concerns related to unwanted ruminations about the past or anticipations of the future they further strengthen their attentional control. The two benefits that flow from this are, first, the evocation during meditation of a more powerful form of the relaxation response and, second, outside of the sessions, an improvement in the ability to avoid being drawn away from present activities.

To repeat, since the crucial process is the act of disengagement, the 'slipping out of the hold of' unwanted, irrelevant or self-defeating thoughts, no great importance attaches to the attentional 'anchor' employed. Benson[2] proposes the silent repetition of the words 'one' or 'out'. We suggest a slightly different focussing technique. The patient is first reminded about the correct style of breathing, getting into a comfortable posture and the rest of the guidelines and is then asked to (silently) say the word 'one' the first time he inhales and to say 'relax' to himself as he breathes out. The next time he breathes in, he is to say (or, better, 'to hear') the word 'two' and, again, 'relax' on breathing out. The general rule, then, is to increase the count one number with each in-breath and to use the word 'relax' on each out-breath.

The attitude of the patient in meditation

It is most important that the patient appreciates the value of holding a tolerant and accepting attitude towards meditation and any difficulties in centering the attention. Hence when the word 'relax' is said, every time he exhales, the patient should take care not to *try* to relax. Any effort towards, or concern with, the degree of relaxation actually achieved should be avoided. The therapist should advise: 'Just say the word and do the counting and let whatever happens happen. Don't *try* to do meditation; just meditate. It is an act, something that is done—not something that will come into being only if you work hard enough. Let your feelings during the execution of this act take care of themselves. Don't approach meditation as a contest in which you might fail through lack of effort.'

Misunderstandings about meditation

Meditation is a simple task and therefore easy

'Count-relax' meditation is a simple technique. It can be taught in one session and most patients find it easy to do and pleasant to experience during the first, therapist-directed practise session.

Expecting to find the same ease of attentional focussing, patients are invariably disappointed when they first try it at home without the expert assistance of the therapist. The complaint most usually mentioned is an inability to stay with the task. Most find that at the start they are easily distracted and sooner or later forget what they should be doing and lose themselves in this, that or the other 'pushy' attention-deflecting thought. The reason for this clinic versus home difference is that in the therapist's office there is an external aid to attentional, here-and-now focussing. This consists of the therapist's voice, presence, and directions as he takes the patient through the first exercise, counting and saying 'relax' aloud in tandem with the patient's silent repetitions, plus suggestions for regular, correct breathing.

A common reaction to distractions is for the patient to become angry with himself ('Damn, I've wandered away again! Why don't I stay with it?'). This, of course, is fruitless; when the patient gets caught in self chastisement he is taken further still from the job at hand. Le Shan's words on this problem are most useful in helping the patient to be patient: 'Treat yourself as if you were a much loved child that an adult was trying to keep walking on a narrow sidewalk'. Most people try the seemingly easy task of meditation only to discover once they try on their own that, in the colourful phrases of an Eastern teacher, they have the 'attention span of a hummingbird' and the 'consciousness of drunken monkey'. It is a good practice to predict and describe the difficulties of distractability before the patient makes his first solo effort and subsequently to reinforce this point at the next meeting. If these reminders are left out, and if the patient is not urged to continue, the 'distractability problem' will lead to an end of meditation training before it has had a chance to do any good.

The therapist's predictions can help to soften the initial disappointment when these difficulties arise.

> 'Here in the clinic, meditation, or, as I have been calling it, attention centering, may have seemed easy to do and pleasant to experience. Tomorrow, at home, when you try to do it on your own it will be anything but easy. The problem will be distraction. All people find this to be so, some more than others. Some people do not get as far as "five" before they veer away from the count-relax meditation technique into tangential con-

cerns and aimless reveries, or else get stuck in some round-and-round cycle of stress thoughts and feelings. Well, if that happens, and it is likely to, you'll sooner or later "catch yourself". Just pick up the count and recommence the exercise. At that time check to be sure that you have not deviated from the proper style and rate of breathing, for when you lose the present-centredness, it is more than likely that you will find that you have reverted to the old maladaptive breathing patterns.'

Mistaking the purpose of meditation
The therapist who has had little experience in teaching patients the rationale and techniques of meditation may be surprised at the usual reports from the patient about his first week's attempts. Regardless of how much emphasis is given to the problems of distractability, and the ill-advised tactic of trying to deal with it by attempting to push unwelcome thoughts from the mind, the patient will complain 'I just couldn't get it right. I couldn't make my mind clear—the opposite, if anything. And as hard as I tried I could not relax.' The therapist must challenge the patient's belief that he was sent home to work at achieving a blank mind and perfect tranquillity. The therapist should advise:

> 'Recall the distinction between attention, the "searchlight", and the thoughts and images illuminated by it. Do not try to expel thoughts from the mind. When you "come to" in the middle of a reverie, withdraw your attention and return it to the focussing task. Gradually, as the weeks go by, you will become more skilled at, first, "catching yourself" before you have been "away" for too long and, second, disengaging your attention from these 'traps' and coming back to whatever it is that you wish to have at the centre of your sustained focus. During the two meditation sessions the focus is on "one" (etc.) "relax"; in your everyday life it will be on the meal you are eating, the walk you are taking or whatever it is that is appropriate for that time and that place.' (The 'camel' example cited earlier can be used to show the futility of 'mind clearing'.)

Trying to recapture 'good feelings' of previous meditations
Once a patient becomes practised and acquires some proficiency

at meditation there may come a day when he experiences a deep and refreshing serenity in a particular session. Understandably, he will look forward to a similar 'high' the next time he meditates. When it does not materialise there is a risk that he may engage in misguided efforts to reproduce the sought-after feelings. Typically, he will get the reverse and, in addition, lose touch with the important objective of meditation—learning how to become 'present centred' while keeping free of irrelevant concerns.

The patient can be steered around such problems and misunderstandings by the comparison of meditation with an exercise like jogging. On occasion the act of jogging may be accompanied by an exquisite feeling of peace. Though pleasant, such a mood is not the justification for jogging. The benefits of jogging come from keeping the heart operating at or above a particular rate for a certain number of minutes. There are days when jogging will be more like a chore than a pleasure. What counts, though, is not how you feel but what you do. The same can be said about meditation. It would be splendid if you could feel profoundly moved each time you meditate, but the fact of the matter is that you will not. The best advice, therefore, is to take the agreeable reactions for what they are, the by-products and not the basic goals of meditation. Training the attention and, indirectly, worry and arousal control are the reasons for engaging in the regular, systematic use of meditation. In addition to being reminded not to try to 'get rid' of 'bad' thoughts the patient should be counselled against chasing after good feelings. The more they are pursued the more elusive they will become.

Meditation is successful when it culminates in sleep

Some patients believe that sleep is the best outcome of any good meditation session. The reply to this is to note that attentional training stops the instant sleep sets in. If patients have difficulties in staying awake it is a sign that the exercise is being done too late at night or when the patient is too tired. Fighting off sleep will not be as difficult if meditation is done earlier in the evening or before taking on strenuous tasks.

Meditation implies an orientation to life which prohibits thinking of the past or the future

The last of the most common misunderstandings turns on a too-literal interpretation of the advice that the patient should be able to choose a particular thought (or object or activity) on which to focus his attention while meditation. He is also urged to adopt this 'here-and-now' orientation at all other times, whatever the activity. Patients sometimes mistakenly think this is a direction never to consider events from the past or likely future activities. If this misinterpretation occurs it can be corrected by stressing:

> 'It is appropriate every so often to sit down and go over the events of the past days or to engage in careful planning for whatever it is that you wish to accomplish in the times to come. Notice, though, that I am distinguishing the decision to put aside time to review and plan from the inappropriate, intrusive recall of the past and imaginings about the future when you should—and wish—to be fully attentive to the experiences of the present. Thus, when it is time for bed then it is time to sleep and not to plot, plan and rehearse all of your tomorrows.'

Recording meditation

Throughout the book the issues of compliance and cooperation have been reiterated. They arise once again in the use of meditation therapy. Records from a University of New South Wales Clinic sample of more than 100 patients indicate that unless special steps are taken, patients will fail to keep up with the twice-daily schedule. Many reasons are given ('I have my hands full all day looking after the kids') but there is no schedule so busy that the patient cannot find the few minutes each day for meditation. To change good intentions into good practice the therapist must take his role as motivator seriously. The patient's intellectual understanding of the principles and aims of meditation is no guarantee that he will follow this up with daily practise.

Exhortation and reminders can help, but not as much as having the patient record his efforts, or lack thereof, each day. Patients can be given sheets like the one pictured as Fig. 11.1 and asked to fill one out every morning and afternoon. If meditation is done on Monday morning but not in the afternoon/evening then 'Yes' should be circled for the former and 'No' for the latter. Patients are also requested to put down the number of minutes for each meditation and whether it was 'easy' or 'difficult'.

At the start of each week's session the record sheet should be reviewed with the patient. In addition to serving as a useful

FIGURE 11.1 A meditation record sheet

Full Meditations

	Date	a.m.	Duration	Rating	p.m.	Duration	Rating
Monday	6/8	yes no	10 mins	difficult	yes no	20 mins	difficult
Tuesday	7/8	yes no			yes no	20 mins	easy
Wednesday	8/8	yes no	20 mins	difficult	yes no	20 mins	easy
Thursday	9/8	yes no	15 mins	easy	yes no		
Friday	10/8	yes no	20 mins	easy	yes no	15 mins	easy
Saturday	11/8	yes no	20 mins	difficult	yes no	20 mins	difficult
Sunday	12/8	yes no	20 mins	easy	yes no	20 mins	easy

motivational aid, home recording can serve as a focus for discussion. It may be revealed that a 20 minute requirement is too demanding for especially 'restless' patients. The sensible response in these circumstances is to suggest that the patient do less than 20 minutes and to add a small amount each day or two. To start, meditation may last only a minute or two. As soon as possible, however, the patient should begin to increase this at his own pace until he reaches the 20 minute mark.

No matter how much patients improve as a result of meditation therapy, there will be a temptation to neglect the daily recordings. At first the record sheet may only be filled in on the day the patient is to meet with the therapist. This is unacceptable. Retrospective recordings are of little value, but more important than the inaccuracies they may contain, failure to maintain daily recording predicts a decline in the number and duration of actual sessions. At first the effects of missing practise may not be felt, but within a week or two worry will begin to climb back to pretreatment levels. Meditation is a *control* technique and *not a cure* for worry. To drive home this point I have found it useful to tell patients about Benson's work with hypertensive patients. Within weeks of beginning meditation Benson's patients had moved from the borderline-high blood pressure range down to the normal range. Normal readings were also registered in non-meditation periods of the day. Overall, those were significant and gratifying changes, but Benson was at pains to have it understood that meditation therapy did not produce a 'cure'. Those few hypertensive patients who stopped meditating showed a return to the initial pre-treatment levels within four weeks. The lesson is:

meditation supports the mental and physical gains of therapy and recording supports meditation.

Problems and special techniques

Noise control

If patients are very sensitive to noise they may never get past the distractable stage for as long as there are audible changes going on around them. The experienced meditator should be able to cut out the sounds around him, but the novice is unlikely to be able to. A number of options can be considered. A simple one is to change the time of meditation to, say, early in the day before the rest of the household has got up. The patient may find it easier to schedule meditation periods when the children are asleep or at school. The working person may have to get up earlier to have quiet for meditaiton. An associate, Dr Wayne Wardman, recommends the use of cottonwool in the ears before starting practice sessions. This reduces the loudness of the noises and provides the bonus of an amplification of the sounds of breathing. With cottonwool in the ears, the sound of your breathing becomes quite noticeable. It is a pleasant, soothing sound not unlike that of the waves washing in and out on the beach. There are clinical reports that any regular, soft, hissing sound, by itself, can act as a valuable aid to relaxation.

'Outside' meditation

If the patient becomes used to particular aids or a carefully arranged environment in which to meditate the chances are that he will find he is unable to meditate in places where less than ideal conditions prevail. Which is to say, he may only be able to centre his attention when conditions are absolutely perfect for centering his attention! To prevent this failure of generalisation patients can be asked to practise additional centering exercises at other times. These 'mini-meditations' can be done at any time of the day as follows. With the eyes open, the patient takes one deep effortful breath, and then establishes an easy, moderate rate of breathing. When he has done this, as he should within a few seconds, he begins the (silent) count-relax technique, going from 'one' to 'ten'. At the end of the tenth breath one mini-meditation has been completed. These can be done ten or more times each day. At least a few of them should be programmed during times of boredom or mild stress (such as when washing the dishes or walking past a pub). Mini-meditations, too, should be recorded on a meditation record sheet like the one shown in Fig. 11.2, and any problems discussed with the therapist.

FIGURE 11.2 A mini-meditation record sheet

Mini Meditations

	Date	a.m.	p.m.
Monday	6/8	√√√√√	√√√√√√
Tuesday	MM	√√√√√√	
Wednesday	8/8	√√√√√√	√√√√
Thursday	9/8	√	√√
Friday	10/8	√√√√√√√√	√√√√√√
Saturday	11/8	√√√√√√	√√
Sunday	12/8	√√√√√√√	√√√√√√√√√

Other modifications

The attention-centering method described earlier for use with most patients may not be ideal for all (whether major or mini-meditations). For the patient who is excessively concerned with achievement, the counting technique may be counterproductive if it leads him to dwell upon how far he got yesterday and how much further he hopes to go today, or to gauge how far he is from the 'goal' of completion. All goals are unhelpful in meditation, most of all the goal of 'getting it over with'. When this becomes an intrusive concern, the meditation procedure can be modified. A simple way to cope with these 'achievement' urges is to have the patient count up to '20' (one breath at a time) and then to start over at 'one' the next time he breathes in.

Another problem, although uncommon, is found in patients who become so adept at the rote execution of the count-relax sequence that they can give back the greater part of their attentional resources to the usual round of hopes, dreads and stray thoughts. If this is the case, two possible counter-strategies can be employed. If the count-relax procedure has become automatic, then it may be helpful to modify the meditation routine so that the patient is required to make some relatively easy but non-rote computation on each breath. The rule could be: 'Start each sequence at 100 (instead of one) and subtract four (or three) every other breath so that when breathing in the number on successive in breaths would be 100, 96, 93, 89, 86, 82, 79, 75, 72 . . .' On every other breath 'calm' and 'relax' could be alternated.

There are patients who prefer to use their own Sanskrit mantra for attention centering. This should not be discouraged, given that the themes are not depressing, frightening or too exciting. The reason for taking care with the content of the meditation exercise may not be apparent to the patient. It is that imagery associated with highly valued activities (winning a competition or achieving a great personal success) can provoke levels of tension and arousal which are distracting and, ultimately, counterproductive. That is because these scenes or themes capture the control of the attention and not the other way around.

Lastly, the patient may wish to explore the use of an eyes-open (i.e. staring) meditation, although as a rule this is not ideal. The 'pull' of the sighted environment is usually too strong, especially if the person has few skills of attentional control. But what about mini-meditations which are done with the eyes open? First, a major meditation lasts 20 minutes, while a mini-meditation lasts only about a minute. Second, mini-meditations are designed as a supplement to and not a substitute for the two 20-minute sessions. The latter *must* be done if the full benefits of meditation are to be realised. However, when a patient is eager to try visual meditation the following advice can be offered. The same effortless approach should be used as in all other forms of meditation. The person should let his gaze fall and remain upon some object without getting caught up in the intellectual significance or emotional reactions associated with the object. If certain thoughts and feelings do arise spontaneously, that is all right as long as the meditator lets them pass and returns his attention to the object. A certain discipline must be exercised against the urge to 'jump' from thing to thing. But staring at any one thing is fatiguing. Switch to a new object at the beginning of each (slow regular) breath cycle (i.e. about once every ten seconds or so).

All meditating techniques can be supplemented by carefully selected and controlled movements. For example, the hands can be firmly but not rigidly clenched as the patient inhales. The tension thus produced is held for two breaths and released in coordination with that outbreath. When the patient feels a little too 'pent up' to do the standard meditation, a few minutes of combined muscle relaxation plus meditation can be advised. The patient must guard against allowing the increments and decrements in tension to cause an interference with an even, easy breathing cycle.

'Meditation' and meditation for attention centering

It might seem odd or unfortunate that we have said so much about meditation without mentioning spiritual or ethical themes. For much of its history meditation has been intimately tied up with religious or moral ideas. It might be said that their absence in our treatment is proof that we have used the wrong word for our discussion of the control of anxiety. We would not object to this conclusion. Our aim has been to show the connection between attention, thoughts, feelings and behaviour and then to present techniques for the modification of attention, the central process in this system. At the same time, we are aware of the great comfort people derive from participation in the ceremonies of TM or other schools of meditation. Our main point has been that drinkers suffer from anticipatory as well as impact anxiety, depression and anger and therefore that cognitive (i.e. attention) control is a vital element in a programme of therapy.

Hypnosis

We have written a volume on hypnosis, behaviour therapy and the treatment of anxiety and phobias. There we noted the overlap of meditation procedures and hypnosis[27]. We can see some benefit for 'meditation-hypnosis' in the treatment of problem drinking, however, as regards heterohypnosis—with a professional hypnotist and the patient in a recaptive mode—there are serious potential drawbacks. Alcohol treatments, by whatever name, if they are to be successful require active problem solving, skill learning and self-control techniques. Our worries about hypnosis are that until alcoholic patients perceive that their active participation is essential to goal planning and the use of self-change procedures they may be attracted to the ideas of magical cures which are enthusiastically promoted by unqualified 'hypnotherapists'. We tell patients who ask for hypnotherapy that there is no such thing. People get treated in and not by hypnosis. Or as Martin Orne of the University of Pennsylvania challenged: 'Anyone with a modicum of training can learn to hypnotise the 80 per cent or so who are "susceptible", but what', he asked, 'do you do then?' Direct suggestion ('you will never drink again'; 'alcohol will taste vile'; 'you will never want to drink again') does not work. It is possible to use hypnosis to assist 'aversion therapies' (nausea suggestions) but not as therapy itself. It can be used to achieve relaxation but on the whole, the self-control strategies of choice are those with support in data, such as the two we have described.

CHAPTER 12

Relapse Therapy

Relapse therapy or, as we prefer to call it, lapse preparation, is new on the scene. Its arrival was delayed by acceptance of the clinical stereotype of the average alcoholic, the belief being held virtually without question that alcoholics who achieve 'cures' in treatment will soon find their way back to drinking and into the relapse statistics. Alcoholics, like smokers, are considered to be chronic recidivists. Mark Twain, when asked about giving up smoking, replied 'Quitting smoking is easy—I've done it a hundred times'. Drinkers, unlike smokers, are less likely to make hundreds of attempts. What seems like unchallengeable support for this belief in recidivism was given in the figures of Hunt et al. which are repeatedly cited as hard evidence for the ever-present risk—indeed the virtual certainty—of relapse. Hunt and his coworkers[1] outlined the results of a large body of clinical findings from a variety of laboratories summarising the longer term outcomes of patients who had been 'cured' of a variety of 'addictions'. The composite graph showed very similar relapse rates across all of the 'addictive' disorders studied: smoking, heroin use and alcohol abuse. Within 90 days post treatment, 60 to 65 per cent had begun to smoke, use heroin or drink again. By the end of a one-year follow-up assessment the relapse figures were higher still.

Though on the face of it discouraging but convincing, the Hunt et al. data must be treated with some reservations. While they review the drinking behaviour, post 'cure', of a large number of patients, all of the results were taken from studies in which there was but one cessation attempt. It is possible that such relapse statistics over-represent those who have failed at prior 'informal' attempts to end drug problems without seeking professional help. Many drinkers (as well as smokers and other drug abusers) do in fact succeed in achieving their goals with the help of relatives and others in their social network. Thus undue pessimism about the maintenance of treatment gains should be qualified with the reservation that Hunt et al.'s data in all likelihood refer mostly to 'hard core' cases. It is also important to remember that Hunt's data are from groups of patients representing the average outcomes from individuals with diverse problems. Such data do not provide information on the factors linked to relapse in the individual case. Therefore, while the relapse curves should not be dismissed as useless, they must be read carefully. When they are, clinically useful information can be gleaned from them. Most importantly, they tell us that backsliding is most likely to occur in the first 90 days following the termination of successful therapy. That gives the therapist and the patient a reasonably good idea of the post-therapy period requiring extra vigilance.

Before moving on to the details of relapse therapy we should ask what we mean by 'relapse'. We can then examine the practical consequences which follow on from the definition of this term. The two meanings given to 'relapse' are sometimes confused one with the other. The most ominous one is defined by the *Shorter Oxford English Dictionary* as: 'to fall back into wrong doing or error; to fall back into an illness after partial recovery'. This comes closer to the meaning of relapse found in traditional clinical thinking than the second one which is listed under the heading 'lapse' (often used as a synonym for relapse): 'a deviation from one's rule of action; a weak or incautious falling from rectitude; to cause to slip or fall, to draw down'. By the standards of the disease/loss-of-control model any return to drinking is described as a return to 'square one'. This interpretation preserves the first meaning of relapse, but it is a hypothesis rather than a description of reality.

Using the definition of 'lapse' takes us in a different direction. It identifies the problem as the probability of 'slips' or 'falls' as items for the end-of-treatment agenda. It acknowledges the possibility of deviations from the optimal state achieved in therapy without giving the sense of foreboding carried by 'relapse'. If the distinction is kept clear then 'lapse' encourages us to seek a reason for the slip without implying that all post-treatment problems with alcohol require that the whole process of therapy be started anew (with the grim corollary that this can only begin, if it ever does, once the relapsed drinker has been forcibly restrained from further drinking).

Another serious criticism of the word 'relapse' (which when used as it usually is is closer in meaning to 'collapse') is that it singles out drinking—or the 'addictions' in general—as having a less sure prognosis than other psychological problems. This is a mistake. The psychiatric literature is replete with evidence of recurring. depression, multiple episodes of agoraphobia, obsessive-compulsive problems that wax and wane, and behaviour-change programmes for schizophrenics which work well in hospital settings but fail to generalise to home or work environments when the patient is discharged.

Increasingly it is recognised that generalisation of good results from therapy to post treatment must be planned for and not assumed. Forms of 'lapse' training have been suggested for ex-agoraphobics[1] and treated schizophrenics and their families.[2] Increasingly programmes are being considered for the challenges that face the ex-problem drinker after the conclusion of therapy. There can be no justification for leaving him in a naive state about the difficulties which may arise after successful therapy. The cliché 'forewarned is forarmed' is particularly apt in this context. Possible problems must be discussed with the patient prior to the termination of therapy.

The decision to include lapse management at the end of therapy provokes critical questions: 'Isn't lapse management, then, simply a continuation of therapy, and if it is, why give it a special name? Why draw distinctions?' The reason for distinguishing lapse therapy from the first stage of therapy is that it asks the patient to anticipate possible 'failures' and to prepare for them. Given that an essential component of any positive clinical change is the restoration of hope, the therapist's task at this point is particularly demanding. Lapse therapy must leave the patient's confidence intact while at the same time preparing him for the possibility of slips. It is most important that the patient be dissuaded from assuming that progress in therapy has been fragile and temporary simply because he is being asked to make prudent precautions. A precondition for the inclusion of lapse therapy in any treatment progrmame is confidence in its value. This requires that three questions be answered: (a) 'Can the probability of slips be predicted with greater than chance accuracy?'; (b) 'If "yes", can steps be taken beforehand to reduce the probability of slips?' and (c) 'Is recovery possible once a slip or two have occurred?'

To take up the first question, we have seen that difficulties are most likely to occur in the first 90 days after the conclusion of treatment. Cummings, Gordon and Marlatt[3] examined extensive descriptive data carefully in search of the precipitants of lapses. They assessed 311 drinkers, smokers, gamblers and the obese. For the ex-drinkers (the data from the other disorders will not be considered here) resumption of problem drinking was linked to:

negative emotional states	38 per cent
interpersonal conflict	18 per cent
social pressures	18 per cent
testing personal control	9 per cent
	83 per cent

The findings match those reported by other investigations[4] and show that between 80 and 90 per cent of the cases of recidivism are tied to identifiable and predictable situations in the patient's life. The link between relapses and certain events is not in doubt, but besides conveying information of this sort to the drinker, more can be done. By the end of therapy the patient will have covered the principles and skills of cognitive restructuring and meditation (to cope with negative emotional states) and assertive behaviour (adaptive ways of managing interpersonal conflict). These skills are intended for combined use and are not presented as compartmentalised and unrelated areas of self management. If used appropriately they can, together with careful screening, accurate assessment, counselling, incentive modification therapy (where applicable) and relaxation techniques help the patient to his initial success. Lapse preparation, the final and most important step in treatment, is designed to help the patient prepare for high risk situations and, if he falters, to enable him to recover from slips. At this time data on the preferred ways to manage recovery from lapses are limited, but sufficient nevertheless to guide the steps which can be taken to facilitate recovery.

We began this chapter with the remark that relapse/lapse therapy is relatively new on the scene. It would be immensely helpful if the existing data could be reduced to a unified set of underlying rules to guide the processes, but what we have instead is a potpourri of useful procedures. This is not intended as a derogatory remark. Lapse therapy is only now coming to the attention of clinician-researchers, thanks mainly to the work of Alan Marlatt. To start, the best guide to the practitioner is the obvious one of fitting the procedure to the patient. The blunderbuss strategy, that of using every potentially helpful technique 'in order to be sure', could be counter-productive in that it risks reducing the drinker's cooperation with the programme and the acquisition of the needed skills. We will here cover the most promising procedures.

Information

We have heard colleagues (most often sociologists) state their opposition to the very idea of relapse/lapse therapy because they consider it potentially counterproductive. This fear derives from 'labelling theory' which says that to give serious attention to lapses is to edge the drinker towards them. The objection is that the underlying message that the patient will hear is 'I [the therapist] have no confidence in your promises or in the stability of your newly won gains'. A companion fear is that patients may take any mention of future lapses as the therapist's belief that 'relapse' is normal and to be expected. The other extreme is the belief that successful treatment confers an immunity upon him (and virtually all want to believe this).

We know from data already discussed that there is a definite link between interpersonal disputes, negative mood states, pressure to drink and the occurrence of lapses. Failure to attach importance to lapse training is akin to denying the possibility of these singly or collectively confronting the patient in the future. Information must be given and the starting point could be the stress-diathesis model developed by Meehl,[5] mentioned earlier. While the diatheses are not easily changed—if they can be modified at all—the positive message is that by themselves they do not constitute a clinical condition. It takes stressful situations, improperly managed, to potentiate the diathesis/vulnerability into an active psychological problem. The stress-diathesis model directly contradicts the claim that abusive drinking is entirely a physiochemical disorder. When a psychological problem is given an exclusively biological explanation (genetic or disease) patients so instructed cope less well than those who are taught about the ways in which learning and the environment affect the disorder.

Problem solving and high risk situations

Chaney, working with Marlatt and others[6] set out to counter feelings of 'learned helplessness' with the aim of preparing the patients to take corrective, adaptive actions when pressures to drink reappeared. Patients in a hospital treatment programme were randomly assigned to one of three groups. The patients had a mean age of 45 and a mean drinking duration of 17 years. The three groups were:

(a) *skills training* Sixteen situations associated with the categories of high risk (see above) were presented to the patients who were asked to respond orally to these situations (for example, from the frustration and anger category: 'your employer criticises you without good reason'). Eight sessions were run in all. At the start the patients were first given basic instructions on stepping back from maladaptive reactions and then practice in generating more reasonable reactions ('what would you say or do?') and assessing the likely consequences of each. Therapists modelled (performed) a range of effective reactions and patients then rehearsed the preferred reaction and received feedback.
(b) *discussion only group* Patients in this group spent as much time talking about the same high risk challenges but the emphasis was dynamic in orientation and centred on the feelings experienced. Problem solving, modelling, rehearsal and feedback were omitted.
(c) *no treatment control group* These patients were given the usual inpatient ('orthodox') therapy.

Following discharge all patients were monitored on a regular basis for one year. Overall, the skills patients did best. The discussion and control groups did not differ significantly from each other. Those in the skills group had approximately 1/6 the number of days drunk, 1/5 the amount of alcohol consumed and about 1/8 the number of drinking days compared with the other two groups. Actual practice, rehearsal, 'as if' instruction (modelling) and feedback were much more useful than having the patients discuss the kinds of feelings they would experience in identical situations. (Which of the four major components applied to the skills group was the most important cannot be estimated. Our guess is that role playing and modelling are crucial.)

The general conclusions from this well-planned study are that patients must: (a) be made aware of high risk situations; (b) consider and practice different and more adaptive alternatives from the usual sequences (get angry, get depressed, get drunk); and (c) in so doing learn that regardless of their habitual responses in the past, the future does not have to be burdened by such failures.

Cue-exposure therapy

In a novel comparison of two quite different disorders, Rankin and his colleagues[7] liken the urges to drink commonly reported by problem drinkers to the reactions experienced by those with obsessive compulsive disorders: 'Frequently, both compulsions and addictions are so powerful that family or work responsibilities are ignored'. From this similarity they reasoned that a proven therapy for compulsive behaviours should have potential for application with drinkers. The therapy in question, 'response prevention', confronts the compulsive with the stimulus (i.e. dirt) that typically provokes long spells of ritualistic hand washing which are hypothesised to be anxiety-reducing rituals. Response prevention is perfectly described by its label: the patient in the face of a strong urge to do so, is prevented from executing his compulsive behaviour. Initially this can be done with others present to ensure restraint; by degrees supervisory controls are removed over sessions until the time when the patient is able, unaided, to refrain from the compulsive behaviours. Rankin and his group developed a comparable intervention for problem drinkers.

In their study drinkers in one group were given two drinks of their preferred alcoholic beverage to consume. A third drink was made available after the two priming drinks. The patients were requested to sit in front of the third drink but to resist the urge to have it. In six sessions only one of the severely alcoholic patients took the final drink. To check on the role of actual versus vicarious contact with the drink there was a control group for comparison which received no alcohol. Their task was to visualise the same sequence of events minus any real contact with the drinks. The results were consistent with the experimenters' assumptions. On subjective and objective measures the 'cue-exposure' group showed a significant decrease in 'desire to drink' and a decline in the difficulty in resisting urges. The control subjects showed no changes.

Elsewhere Hodgson and Rankin report on the successful use of cue-exposure with a number of individual cases to protect against lapses.[8] The early results and the theoretical rationale give this simple and ingenious technique a claim to further investigation, but until there are long-term controlled clinical studies corroborating these preliminary findings, cue-exposure must be considered a promising but untested therapy.

The additional comment we wish to make about cue-exposure as a method of lapse prevention centres on the negative reactions which we encountered from the 'abstinence lobby'. In our preliminary proposal we went out of our way to stress our awareness that for some patients any drinking is contraindicated. Accordingly we proposed a controlled clinical investigation of cue-exposure with appropriate screening procedures to ensure that 'vulnerable' patients were not admitted to the study. The sticking point came, as we had feared it would, with our stated intention to give alcohol to problem drinkers. We have heard of other clinical researchers in North America encountering considerable resistance when attempting to obtain referrals and to recruit patients for such therapy. Thus we expect that the work on cue-exposure response prevention therapy will proceed slowly in the forseeable future.

Stimulus-control therapy

All commercially available alcoholic drinks have a distinctive taste and smell. In the experience of the patient across years of heavy drinking these stimuli, plus those linked to the distinctive labels and containers of a particular kind and brand of alcohol, are repeatedly associated with the effects of alcohol, both positive and negative. The positive effects occur earlier and are more likely to be conditioned to the smell, taste and look of the drink. That is the theory. The evidence points to the existence of learned associations of this kind and their relation to relapse. In heavy drinkers physiological responses occur to the sight of a specific container and the taste and/or smell of the drinker's preferred drink.[9] Reports of cravings for drinks have been correlated with these physical and psychological reactions, opening up the possibility that long after abstention one-time problem drinkers may experience conditioned withdrawal reactions when they next encounter the smell of an alcoholic drink or actually have a drink or two.

One recent study of particular interest to clinicians showed that 'dry alcoholics' and others still receiving treatment salivated significantly more to the smell of their favourite alcoholic beverage than non-problem drinkers. Moreover, the smell alone significantly increased the desire to drink alcohol in the 'dry alcoholics' as well as in the patients receiving treatment. The patient who showed the greatest salivation and swallowing to the smell of his drink was the only one to consume the drink. The authors of this study wrote of him: 'Drinking in the test situation flatly contradicted the patient's prior statements to the effect that he could handle situations where alcohol was present' (which he had not had to face since entering treatment). The session was terminated immediately and the patient's therapist used this to document the potency of alcohol related cues. Despite a prior history of resisting treatment the patient then participated actively in relapse-prevention training, was cooperative in the Alcoholics Anonymous programme and willingly took disulfiram.

Our own clinical trials have suggested another way to employ smell cues as a means of protecting against the risk of lapses coming about through exposure to conditioned salivary responses and the concomitant desire to drink. Borrowing from laboratory extinction procedures first used by Pavlov and, of late, by behaviour therapists using exposure procedures to treat phobic anxiety, we have used three 5-minute exposure trials over five sessions to reduce the salivary response and, with it, the subjective 'desire to drink'. On the first trials patients are given cottonwool to smell that has been soaked in the type of drink with the highest risk factor. The trials finish with the patient holding and smelling the alcoholic drink.

A variation is to have the patient practice meditation or relaxation for 15 minutes prior to presentation of the smell in conjunction with imagined recall and visualisation of typical drinking locales. (Exposure to imaginal cues alone is of little value.) It is an open question as to how the extended smell-exposure trials work to attenuate the 'pull' of alcohol. Conditioned inhibition, enhanced self-confidence, or, simply, learning how to 'resist' the conditioned cravings are possible explanations to be explored further.

There are obvious affinities between cue-exposure and stimulus-control therapies. The intent is identical: to allow the ex-problem drinker to be exposed to the temptations which sooner or later are likely to come his way after the close of therapy. If all other things are equal, then proposals for the adoption of stimulus-control therapy should produce fewer objections in those of a conservative bent because it does not include the actual consumption of alcohol.

Other approaches to relapse therapy

The third question posed at the start of this chapter still remains: is recovery possible once a serious lapse occurs? The short answer is that there is no scientific evidence to answer the question. One method is the scheduling of 'booster' sessions. No one would quibble with this suggestion, though it does not answer the question. From the evidence, drinkers with social supports and/or residential and occupational stability stand the best chance of coping. It has also been suggested that patients be asked to consider 'life-style modification', but finding out what that should be and how it can best be brought about are tasks still before us. Social support would appear to be the key factor. Social support can be found within a positive relationship with spouse or family and the assistance of a support network specifically concerned with maintaining clinical gains or reestablishing them. In many respects the model has come from Alcoholics Anonymous (AA) and though we have some reservations about its ideas and methods, it is an influence to be reckoned with. On a practical level it has, and no doubt will continue to have, a major following.

Alcoholics Anonymous

One of the most successful outcomes in the annals of alcohol treatment studies was recorded in the aversion therapy (i.e. incentive modification) treatments by Le Mere, Voegtlin and their team in the 1950s (see Chapter 9). An often overlooked result from their work was the higher success rates attained by the drinkers who also joined abstinence societies. AA is the best known of these societies and the one that attracts the overwhelming majority of referrals from counsellors. It has recorded dramatic successes, but even applying the most favourable estimates the success rates do not justify the present general practice of automatic recommendation of AA as the form of relapse prevention. Some benefit from AA contact, others do not. Who are the drinkers most likely to accept referrals to AA and who are the drinkers best suited to AA's methods and philosophy? Addressing these questions Edwards concedes that 'it is always difficult to predict who will and who will not find AA helpful'. AA does not publish such data but informal estimates suggest that drinkers in the upper ranges of alcohol dependence are the best candidates. Problem drinkers who rank lower in dependence are less likely to agree to the unbending insistence on absolute alcohol avoidance which is a founding principle of AA

As AA is and will continue to be urged upon problem drinkers, a short outline of its programme in action will give the counsellor an idea of what actually happens at the meetings. This information will provide a basis for judging whether there would be a 'fit' between AA and his patient, and will give the patient some idea of what will be expected of him. Not all AA groups have the same composition and emphasis (apart from the universal adherence to an abstinence regimen) and there are differences from country to country. The social constitutions of groups will differ and the drinker may wish to attend a number of different groups before settling with one.

AA in operation

The basic philosophy of AA is encoded in the famous 12 steps.

1. We admit we were powerless over alcohol—that our lives had become unmanageable.
2. Came to believe that a Power greater than ourselves could restore us to sanity.
3. Made a decision to turn our will and our lives over to the care of God as we understood Him.
4. Made a searching and fearless moral inventory of ourselves.
5. Admitted to God, to ourselves, and to another human being the exact nature of our wrongs.
6. Were entirely ready to have God remove all these defects of character.
7. Humbly asked him to remove our shortcomings.
8. Made a list of all persons we had harmed and became willing to make amends to them all.

9. Made direct amends to such people wherever possible, except when to do so would injure them or others.
10. Continued to take personal inventory and when we were wrong promptly admitted it.
11. Sought through prayer and meditation to improve our conscious contact with God as we understood him, praying only for knowledge of His will for us and power to carry that out.
12. Having had a spiritual awakening as the result of these steps we tried to carry this message to alcoholics and to practice these principles in all our affairs.

AA meetings are attended by varying numbers of people, from a small group up to a hundred or more. Some of them will have been members for years and others will be newly in attendance. The chairman for the evening will be seated at the front of the room with the one or two people who have agreed to tell their stories. The chairman opens the proceedings by giving his first name (no surnames are ever used) and his 'condition': 'Good evening, my name is Phillip; I am an alcoholic'. He then recites the AA preamble:

> 'Alcoholics Anonymous is a fellowship of men and women who share their experience, strength and hope with each other that they may solve their common problem and help others to recover from alcoholism. The only requirement for membership is a desire to stop drinking. There are no dues or fees for AA membership, we are self-supporting through our own contributions. AA is not allied with any sect, denomination, politics, organisation or institution; does not wish to engage in any controversy, neither endorses nor opposes any causes. Our primary purpose is to stay sober and help other alcoholics achieve sobriety.'[10]

Next the speakers begin, and tell of the development of their drinking problems from first contact to 'rock bottom' experiences: ' ". . . and my binges remained one nighters. But they were occurring with alarming frequency . . . and they were growing uglier. One night I barely made it [to my destination], if I'd had to go another fifty feet I'd have collapsed in the gutter. On another occasion I arrived home covered with blood . . . and one night I was in suicidal despair." ' No one is quizzed or coerced to speak.

The meeting ends with the serenity prayer:

'God grant me the serenity
To accept the things I cannot change
The courage to change the things I can
And the wisdom to know the difference.'

AA, then, offers structure, explicit goals, fellowship, an ideology (disease/loss-of-control) and a willingness to persist with backsliders. Edwards writes 'the therapist should always be able, whenever appropriate, to signpost the way to AA'.[11] The key phrase 'whenever appropriate' is still a matter of subjective judgement. At the least it can be said that sobriety requirements do not suit many drinkers. Others may turn away because of the strongly religious feeling as enunciated in the 12 steps. Other concerns are the constant statements of helplessness (Steps 1, 3 and 7) and the implicit but obvious equation of excessive drinking with insanity (Step 2).

Despite our conceptual differences with AA and its defenders (most of the medical profession, psychologists and counsellors) we cannot ally ourselves with the unyielding attitude of some behavioural clinicians who scorn AA as, in every way, a barrier to progress. For some problem drinkers, perhaps not many, it may be the only way to overcome their difficulties.

Conclusion

In 1986 Torrey[12] pointed out that at the start of this decade there were more than 250 varieties ('brands') of therapy in practice for problem drinkers, including the behavioural therapies (for example, aversion therapy) and cognitive therapies (for example, meditation, cognitive restructuring, Gestalt therapy and phenomeno-structural therapy). All but a handful of the 250 rely on the personal commitment of founders and followers to support their various claims for clinical value. Torrey asks: 'What are we to make of this chaotic melange?' He cautions against a summary dismissal of the untested and untestable therapies (the majority). All share the four basic active components which have been abstracted from all of the known schools of psychotherapy:

1. a shared worldview;
2. positive personal qualities of the therapist;

3. patient expectations of positive change;
4. an emerging sense of mastery.

Torrey is not arguing for the interchangeability of any one of the therapies with all others. That argument cannot be defended; as one example, we have already seen that taste aversion therapies are superior to shock aversion therapies. The point Torrey wishes to make is that in addition to the active ingredients (the specific properties of a particular therapy), the four 'non-specific' factors play an important supporting-motivating role. They mobilise positive beliefs and help to establish hope in the possibility of change. Of the four we would press the case for 'mastery', not simply as a 'sense' of self-efficacy but as a measurable reality derived from (a) the patient's understanding of alcohol problems and (b) the acquisition of mastery skills for use in stressful situations. The two together are essential. We believe that the two should be combined, beginning with an analysis of the variety of alcohol problems, and the framing of techniques and therapies according to an understanding of what leads to and sustains the person's entrapment in excessive drinking and the problems that accompany it.

'Much remains to be done' and 'more research is needed' are phrases which appear regularly at the close of research reports to do with all manner of psychological problems. Such phrases would do as well here. Papers and books on alcoholism would benefit from such statements in place of the iron-clad certainties, strident accusations and counter-accusations that abound in the discussion of drinking disorders. The risk of getting caught up in these battles is that the combattants will lose sight of the drinker and his problems. The other risk, equally costly in its own way, is that the less committed ideologically will tire of this atmosphere and retreat into the belief that all therapies are equally effective. The facts say otherwise. Ideally what is required is a complete statement of the various processes of the 'alcoholisms'. This would permit the development of reliable guidelines to the selection of the appropriate treatments and an understanding of how they produce positive outcomes. But we are far from that ideal condition and for many years to come the clinician will have to rely on his intuitions as well as on empirically proven treatments. Continued progress will depend on keeping a careful balance between a disciplined scepticism about, and an openness to, new findings. Above all, dialogue must be kept going among the various disciplines. We have been able to write this book because disinterested and talented clinicians and researchers have carried out the work which has formed the basis for our ideas.

APPENDIX A

Canterbury Alcoholism Screening Test (CAST)

		YES	NO
Q1.	Have you been admitted to hospital more than once because of accidents? (By accidents, we mean all types)	☐	☐
Q2.	Have any close family members such as a parent, brother, spouse, or sister, had drinking problems?	☐	☐
Thinking over THE LAST THREE MONTHS:			
Q3.	Do you drink before lunch fairly often?	☐	☐
Q4.	After the first glass or two of alcohol do you ever feel a craving for more?	☐	☐
Q5.	Do you find you are thinking a lot about alcohol?	☐	☐
Q6.	Do you sometimes drink alcohol against your doctor's advice?	☐	☐
Q7.	When you drink a lot of alcohol, do you tend to eat less?	☐	☐
Q8.	In the morning do you sometimes feel that you might be sick (vomit)?	☐	☐
Q9.	Have you found that your hands have been trembling a lot?	☐	☐
Q10.	Have you ever used alcohol to get rid of trembling or the feeling that you might be sick?	☐	☐
Q11.	Have you ever been criticized at work because of your drinking?	☐	☐
Q12.	Do you prefer to drink alone?	☐	☐
Q13.	Do you think you're in worse shape because of your drinking?	☐	☐
Q14.	Do you ever have a guilty conscience about drinking?	☐	☐

Q15.	In order to cut down your drinking, have you ever felt it necessary to limit it to certain occasions or to certain times of the day?	☐	☐
Q16.	Do you feel you should drink less?	☐	☐
Q17.	Do you think that without alcohol you would have fewer problems?	☐	☐
Q18.	When you're upset do you drink alcohol to calm down?	☐	☐
Q19.	Are there times when you'd like to stop drinking?	☐	☐
Q20.	Would you get along better with your spouse/partner/the people you're closest to if you didn't drink?	☐	☐
Q21.	Have you ever deliberately tried to do without any alcohol at all?	☐	☐
Q22.	Have you often been told that your breath smells of alcohol?	☐	☐

Q23. On the average, write in the number you would normally drink in a week:

Beer	**No.**	**Spirits/ Liqueurs**	**No.**	**Sherry**	**No.**
glass/can	☐	nip	☐	glass	☐
large can	☐	bottle (sm) ...	☐	bottle	☐
handle	☐	bottle (lge) ...	☐		
bottle	☐	**Wine**		**Cocktails**	
jugs	☐	glass	☐	glass	☐
flagon	☐	bottle	☐		

CAST SCORE OVERLAY

1. Align score card with boxes and corner marks.

Col. 1	Col. 2	Col. 3	Col. 1	Col. 2	Col. 3	Col. 1	Col. 2	Col. 3
Beer			**Spirits/ Liqueurs**			**Sherry**		
1 ×	☐	= ☐	1 ×	☐	= ☐	1 ×	☐	= ☐
2 ×	☐	= ☐	16 ×	☐	= ☐	14 ×	☐	= ☐
						Cocktails		
2 ×	☐	= ☐	30 ×	☐	= ☐	2 ×	☐	= ☐
			Wine					
4 ×	☐	= ☐	1 ×	☐	= ☐		B ☐☐	÷
6 ×	☐	= ☐	8 ×	☐	= ☐			
8 ×	☐	= ☐						

TOTAL SCORE: ☐

2. Write in the number of 'YES's' for Questions 1–22 in A.
3. Multiply column 1 and column 2 together, write answers in column 3.
4. Add all the numbers in column 3, and write the total in B.
5. If B equals 36 or more for males, 16 or more for females, write 1 in C, otherwise write 0.
6. Add A and C together and write the total in D.

CLINICIAN'S ASSESSMENT (if available). Check for the presence of a palpable liver, Dupuytrens contracture, elevated GGT and elevated AST. If any one or more of these are present, add one point to D.

TEST INTERPRETATION. The CAST is a screening test designed specifically for hospitalised persons over the age of 15 years. It is not intended to be a fully diagnostic instrument. The following scoring system is suggested: 0–2 for a non-problem drinker, and 3 or more to indicate alcohol problems severe enough to warrant a full clinical assessment. If 1 point is added from the Clinician's assessment, raise the cut-off score to 4 or more.

SOURCE. Elvy, G.A. and Wells, J.E. for the Alcohol Research Committee of the North Canterbury Hospital Board's Working Party on Alcohol and Drug Dependence, P.O. Box 1876, Christchurch.

APPENDIX B

Deranged Ingestion: Foundations of Therapy for Alcoholism*

J. CHRISTOPHER CLARKE

School of Psychology, University of New South Wales, Kensington, NSW, Australia

and

JOHN GARCIA

Department of Psychiatry and Psychology, University of California at Los Angeles, Los Angeles, California, USA

Abstract: *Recent investigations of human and animal learning suggest that the conceptualization of alcoholism and its subsequent treatment might be appropriately based on an understanding of learning mechanisms which control feeding behaviour. Perhaps the most significant in this regard is the research concerning taste aversion and food avoidance. This research, particularly that related to modifying the feeding habits of predators and the management of alcoholism in humans by aversive conditioning, is described in detail in this review. The theoretical significance of the prolonged interval between the conditioned stimulus (the food or drink) and the aversive event and the insights that this research has provided on the notion of equipotentiality and generally of different aversive stimuli are discussed.*

Keywords: *Taste aversion; aversion therapy; hedonic valence.*

Although the problems of alcoholism have long been a serious concern of psychotherapists of all persuasions, the success rates from treatment have not been particularly impressive[1,2]. It is just

* Reprinted from *Australian Drug and Alcohol Review* 1986, *5*, 21–27.

as clear that alcoholism exhibits low remission rates when left untreated.[3] If unchecked, it can be physically debilitative, as well as psychologically devastating. Recently, developments in ethology and experimental psychobiology have led to a more complete understanding of ingestive behaviour and its neural mechanisms. In this paper, we will describe these findings and discuss their implications for aversion therapy in the treatment of alcoholism and problem drinking.

The aims, procedures and concepts of aversion therapy can be stated simply. The *goal* is to reduce or eliminate drinking and overeating by one of two basic procedures. The first procedure, classical (Pavlovian) conditioning, provides the patient with a painful or unpleasant stimulus (e.g. electric shock or emetic drug) immediately after the sight, smell and/or taste of the stimulus to be averted. The drink or food is termed the conditioned stimulus (CS) and the aversive event is called the unconditioned stimulus (US). The theory states that after repeated pairings of the conditioned and unconditioned stimuli closely in time, the conditioned stimulus (e.g. whisky, wine, etc), will elicit the response produced by the unconditioned one (e.g. anxiety, nausea). Since the stimulus selected as the CS-to-be (e.g. the whiskey) becomes aversive in itself, behaviours directed at consuming the aversive stimulus are reduced. The second procedure, operant (Skinnerian) conditioning, identifies the *behaviour* (e.g. drinking alcohol) as the problem. Because behaviour is considered to be governed by its consequences, arranging for an aversive outcome to follow the target behaviour should lead to a reduction in that behaviour by sheer punishment. In classical conditioning, the focus is upon changing the incentive value of the conditioned stimulus, while operant conditioning focuses upon eliminating the action that leads to consumption.

Nature of the aversive stimulus

Whichever procedure he adopts, the practicing therapist using these techniques faces an important question. What aversive stimulus should be used? Those who have considered the problem at all have listed primarily two commonsense criteria: safety and unpleasantness.[4] Perhaps the most widely used aversive stimulus has been electric shock, which is usually delivered to the hand or arm during the operant responses of consumption or just after the sight, taste, smell, or thought of a conditioned stimulus to be consumed. Electric shock is both safe and aversive and can be delivered with precise timing and intensity, as required by the traditional conditioning paradigms. With these practical considerations in mind, clinical theorists such as Rachman and Teasdale[5] advocated the replacement of chemicals with electric shock in aversion therapy. Emetic drugs, although less popular, continue to be used to create nausea and a tendency to vomit in association with prohibited drinks or foods. Other workers have used aversive stimuli ranging from loud noises to verbal descriptions of pain and nausea.

This electric approach to the aversive stimulus reflects the profound effects that learning theorists have had upon the practice of clinical behaviour modification. The theory, held almost universally, specifies that aversive stimuli are equipotential and possess transituational generality. If aversive stimuli are equipotential, then one safe aversive stimulus should be as effective as any other equally safe and equally unpleasant stimulus. If an aversive stimulus has transituational generality, then it should be as effective in modifying one behaviour in a given situation as some other behaviour in a different situation. Thus if a rat's bar-pressing or alley-running can be eliminated with the use of contingent electric shock, it is assumed that *any* punishing stimulus, if used at the right intensity, and often enough, can eliminate *any* behaviour or create an aversion to *any* conditioned stimulus in all species. These assumptions of equipotentiality and transituational generality allowed the learning theorist to formulate broad, abstract (preferably mathematical) laws on a relatively restricted set of controlled experiments. They also provided the clinician with a practical basis for choosing convenient and "clean" aversive stimuli, responses, and situations, and brings the problems of selective associations to the forefront.

The interchangeability notion was directly tested in a series of experiments and was found to be invalid. Garcia and Koelling[6] found that when taste and audiovisual conditioned stimuli were paired with an illness unconditioned stimulus induced by lithium injections or x-radiation, rats developed a strong aversion for the taste stimulus but not for the audiovisual one. Conversely, when an electric shock was employed as the unconditioned stimulus the rats avoided the audiovisual conditioned stimulus but not the taste one. Subsequent studies disclosed that the interval between the taste CS and the illness US could be prolonged for minutes, even a few hours and conditioned taste aversions would still develop in one trial; but when the audiovisual CS and shock US were used, delays of greater than 30 seconds tend to disrupt conditioning (except under exceptional circumstances). Just as important for therapy, taste aversions induced by illness generalize to other situations in which the taste conditioned stimulus is encountered, while conditioned responses induced by shock tend to be specific to the situation in which they were established.[7] Nausea proved to be a uniquely effective aversive stimulus for the modification of ingestive behaviour.

Aversions acquired for the taste of a toxic meal through a selective learning mechanism are ubiquitous phenomena in the animal kingdom[8] and have attracted scientific attention since the time of Darwin because of their obvious implications for natural selection and species survival[9,10].

Taste-illness aversions in humans

Taste-illness aversions are ubiquitous in human populations as well. After Wilson and Davison[11] proposed that the selective nature of learning has important implications for therapy in humans as well as laboratory rats, it was empirically demonstrated that, as is the case with laboratory rats, a nausea unconditioned stimulus was more effective than a shock one in reducing intake of beverages in college students[12] and more recently in excessive drinkers[13]. Bernstein[14] reported that children under treatment for neoplastic diseases developed conditioned taste aversions specifically for the flavour of an ice cream consumed prior to their chemotherapy despite their cognitive awareness that the resultant nausea was due to the injected drug and not to the flavoured ice cream. Furthermore, these children also tended to dislike or avoid any food that had been eaten several hours before treatment. Neither prior experience with the beneficial food nor prior experience with the toxic illness produced by the toxins prevented the acquisition of a taste aversion in Bernstein's children. The same situation was obtained in laboratory rats[15] and in captive coyotes and wolves[16,17].

The human being's cognitive attribution of cause and effect has surprisingly little effect upon the unpleasant quality which accrues to taste stimuli after a bout of nausea.[18] In a recent study conducted at the Royal North Shore Hospital in Sydney (Clarke, Fisher, Levy, Tebbutt, unpublished manuscript) *adult* patients receiving chemotherapy for serious cancer problems showed the same reactions as Bernstein's children. Pleasant but innocuous tastes consumed prior to the onset of chemotherapy induced malaise lead to a significant reduction in the "pleasantness" ratings of foods or fluids which the patients knew were merely correlated with and not the cause of their malaise. To prove that the pairings of taste and malaise was critical, control groups were made up of other volunteers who also had chemotherapy and the tastes but on separate days. In these individuals there was no change in the attractiveness of the ingested substances.

Mechanisms of aversion

The aversive unconditioned stimulus in conditioned flavour aversions appears to be an activation of brain stem mechanisms that facilitate emesis[19]. Basically, toxins appear to serve as the aversive stimulus in two ways. The first is by peripheral gastric or intestinal irritation which activates central emetic mechanisms via the vagus nerve. Subdiaphragmatic vagotomy blocks both the vomiting reflex[20] and the taste aversion[20] induced by irritation of the stomach with copper sulfate. The second is through blood-borne toxins which stimulate the chemoreceptors of the area postrema which have projections to the emetic system. Vagotomy will not block vomiting,[21] nor the taste aversions[19] induced by intravenous injections of copper sulfate directly into the circulatory system.

Although we have focused mainly on the negative (aversive) action of the mechanisms, they may act in the positive (appetitive) direction also. Arbitrary flavours gain preference when they are paired with recuperation from thiamine deficiency corrected by intraperitoneal injections[22,23] or paired with recovery from intraperitoneal-injected apomorphine[24]. It has also been shown that glucose tastes pleasant when blood sugar is low and unpleasant when blood sugar is high[25]. Therefore, it appears that the vascular route is involved in palatability adjustment in both directions. Also, animals will eat until the stomach is full and when a portion of the food is withdrawn from the stomach, they will compensate by eating an equivalent amount.[26,27] Apparently, gastric signals supply the motive to eat and to stop eating[28], and vagotomy will disrupt these signals.[29,30] Thus, it appears that the vagal route is also involved in appetitive (positive) as well as aversive (negative) reactions.

A question yet to be answered concerns the critical response which must be evoked for tastes to be aversively conditioned. Emesis is an obvious candidate. However strong taste aversions can be produced in rats and they are unable to vomit. A "best guess" at this stage is that nausea is critical if an enduring change is to take place. In a recent experiment Clarke and Hayes[31] created significant decrease in the reactions of volunteers from whom verbally induced nausea was effective. Motion sickness initiated by vestibular and visual stimulation can elicit vomiting and will induce flavour aversions in humans[12,32] and in rats[33] but the neurological and humoral pathways for this particular unconditioned stimulus are not yet clearly defined. Psychological trauma and physiological injury will also trigger emesis. Suffice to say, any agent that produced nausea and vomiting will also produce a conditioned flavour aversion. In fact, the conditioned flavour aversion appears to be a more sensitive behavioural index for emetic mechanism activation than the vomiting reflex itself, since aversions can be established by doses too small to initiate vomiting. On the other hand, vomiting and aversions are obviously related functionally: the acute vomiting reflex ejects poisoned ingesta from the stomach, while the chronic flavour aversions can be considered the most sensitive member of a complex hierarchy of visceral malaise symptoms, which includes, in rough ascending order to dose, anorexia, listlessness, nausea, vomiting, retching, unconsciousness, and death.

Taste stimuli are the most effective conditioned stimuli in flavour aversion conditioning by virtue of their direction projection to the nucleus of the tractus solitarius which is an integral part of the brain stem emetic anatomy[34]. Other food stimuli can become effective if accompanied by taste during the conditioning process. For rats and probably other mammals, odour alone is a weak conditioned stimulus when paired with illness. If odour and taste are combined into a compound conditioned stimulus and followed by illness, odour becomes a very strong stimulus when tested alone in extinction and is particularly effective if it remains in compound with taste[15]. Similarly in birds, visual food stimuli are weak when presented alone, but when combined with a taste conditioned stimulus and followed by an illness unconditioned stimulus, visual cues gain a strong capacity to inhibit ingestion in their own right.[35,36] In other words, the taste element synergistically potentiates weaker stimulus elements of that compound CS called drink; taste does not overshadow or block these weaker elements during the acquisitioned process as traditional conditioning theory would predict.

Taste aversion and traditional conditioning theory

There have been a number of attempts to incorporate taste aversion data into traditional learning formats. Garcia and Koelling[6] felt compelled to admit that common elements in the time-intensity patterns of CS-US stimulation might favour some associations (i.e. buzzer-shock or taste-illness) but not the converse arrangements (i.e. buzzer-illness or taste-shock). Wilson and Davison[11] also suggested that topographical compatibility of conditioned and unconditioned stimuli might facilitate aversive conditioning. Testa and Ternes[37] provide the most detailed defence of the topographical position, arguing that a taste lingers internally in the abdomen, making their association likely; in a similar vein, both audiovisual stimuli and electric foot shock are referred to the external environment, facilitating their association.

However a detailed review of the accumulated evidence does not support the topographical view. When taste in the mouth is the conditioned stiimulus, shock to the mouth is no more effective than shock to the foot[38]. Lingering shocks programmed to mimic illness are no more effective than square wave shock pulses in the productiion of taste aversions[39]. On the other hand, when nausea is the unconditioned stimulus the intitial taste of an ephemeral substance completely changed or drowned out by salivary and digestive processes is an effective conditioned stimulus[39]. Postingestional stimulation, which is closer in locus and time to the ultimate nausea, is not an effective conditioned stimulus[40]. Nausea is an effective unconditioned stimulus whether it is induced by an ingested toxin or by rotation of the environment around the subject[12]. Finally, as we discussed above, taste will potentiate food cues. An environmental odour alone is a weak conditioned stimulus for illness, but if the rat drinks a tasty solution in the presence of that same environment odour, the odour now becomes a powerful conditioned stimulus even though its topographical features are unchanged.[41,42]

Since operant (Skinnerian) conditioning stresses the immediate effects of reinforcement upon responses, taste-illness conditioning does not fit comfortably in that format either. It is not a behaviour modification process based upon the association of eating responses with the contingent punishment of illness. It is an incentive modification process operating over long temporal intervals, primarily upon taste, and secondarily upon other food related stimuli. The taste conditioned stimulus gains some of the noxious properties of the nausea unconditioned stimulus and also becomes unpalatable in its own right. Thus a tasty substance, which once attracted and reinforced approach responses, will elicit signs of disgust and reinforce avoidance responses after pairing with illness. Consider the types of responses developed by a variety of animals upon encountering an averted food. After a single pairing of hamburger and illness, hungry coyotes buried or urinated on fresh hamburger. After a single meal of venison treated with lithium, a cougar walked away from untained venison, gingerly shaking its paws. After one or two meals of prey flesh paired with illness, predators will even inhibit their attacks upon living prey. Hawks retreat from mice[35]. Coyotes slink away from lambs with their tails tucked between their legs.[16] Wolves posture submissively before a sheep as if it were a dominant wolf.[17] This behaviour, which would appear grossly abnormal and pathological for hungry predators were the etiology unknown, arises out of the conflict induced when a familiar food becomes a disgusting, inedible object.

Clinical studies

Emetic drugs have been employed as the aversive stimulus in the treatment of alcoholism for many decades. Lemere and Voegtlin[43] treated more than four thousand patients in a program of such scope and care that it must be considered a major work in the field of aversion therapy. The patients were asked to taste (but not drink) whiskey and, shortly afterward, emetic drugs were administered to produce nausea and vomiting. Twenty or fewer such trials were held over a ten-day period. At the end of one year, they reported a total abstinence rate of 60%. Of those patients who returned for additional booster sessions, the abstinence rate was

90%. Unfortunately, it is not possible to relate these impressive rates solely to the aversive procedures used since other forms of therapy were also employed. Sanderson and his co-workers[44] gave alcoholics succinylcholine chloride (anectine) following the consumption of a preferred alcohol beverage. The patients recorded a feeling of terror and panic in response to the anectine but in spite of the obvious aversiveness of this procedure, success rates of below 20% were recorded, and the data indicated that even the few successes were probably due to other factors. The differences in effectiveness of these two studies may be due to the fact that fear induced by any procedure is primarily associated with the treatment situation, while the nausea induced by an emetic drug causes the target beverage to become unpalatable.

Despite the early successes of Lemere and Voegtlin[43], the use of nausea as the aversive stimulus declined, probably because electric shock was considered safer and could be delivered with the temporal precision required by the traditional paradigms of conditioning. However, under the impetus of taste aversion conditioning, the efficacy of nausea in the treatment of alcoholism has been reconsidered.[4,40,45] Recently, Mellor and Revusky[see 32] employed lithium as the emetic agent in the treatment of twenty-five alcoholics. The subjects were unemployed males with histories of alcohol dependence admitted into a psychiatric hospital while exhibiting tremor, delirium, or seizures; such patients are considered poor risks for treatment rehabilitation. The abstinence rate six months after treatment was 36% (47% if eight patients who did not develop sickness symptoms are excluded). By comparison, an equivalent group of patients given calcium carbimide, a dizzying deterrent like antabuse, had an abstinence rate of only 12%. Mellor and White[32] treated ten subjects (eight males and two females) admitted to the hospital under circumstances similar to those described above. The patients were given alcohol and then rotated in a swivel chair to produce motion sickness. Two patients habituated to the motion treatment, but the remaining eight exhibited severe malaise during each of the twelve treatment trials. Six of the eight subjects tried alcohol during the six-month follow-up period and four of these exhibited aversions to the alcoholic drinks they sampled. The aversion was sufficient to deter two subjects from further drinking. But one subject switched to an unfamiliar drink (vodka and orange juice) which was not aversive and the other subject continued to drink despite nausea and vomiting until the aversion was extinguished. (These "treatment failures" serve to illustrate two principles of taste-illness conditioning: the conditioned aversion is specific to the taste CS, and it can be extinguished with repeated unreinforced trials.)

The work by Cannon et al.[13] referred to earlier is entirely consistent with these findings. Some male alcoholics were given painful (but harmless) electric shock while others were made ill with a malaise producing drug following the taste of certain alcoholic beverages. At six-month follow-up the malaise group were more improved than the shock group.

Conclusions

In conclusion, animal studies from Garcia's laboratory show that tastes associate preferentially with malaise. From this was deduced a number of directions concerning the appropriate use of aversion therapy for problem drinking. Laboratory and clinical data with humans support these recommendations. However, more points deserve emphasis. The first is that it is not aversiveness per se that is crucial. In the aforementioned (and highly criticized) report of Sanderson et al.[44] the alcoholics were told only that something unpleasant would follow the presentation of the alcohol. In fact the curare-like drug employed caused total, temporary paralysis. (The subjects had to be respirated.) Afterwards the alcoholics said that they had been "terrified"—some felt that they were dying. Undoubtedly the treatment was aversive—but it did not change the hedonic valence of the tastes paired with the nightmare "therapy". Second, when a given alcoholic substance is paired with the nausea agent (whether drug-induced, verbally triggered or brought on by "motion sickness") such changes in palatability that occur will accrue to the taste of the targeted substance. Thus patients can not be expected to develop aversions to alcohol but to a particular beverage. If a patient drinks, let us say, whiskey and wine to excess it must not be assumed that if an aversion is (deliberately) induced to wine that similar changes will occur to all other alcoholic beverages. Third, although we have been using the term "taste aversions" what is meant is not merely that the targeted taste (of the alcoholic beverage) is rendered less attractive. That outcome by itself would be trivial. Indeed alcoholics often report that they don't especially care for the taste of the substance which they regularly abuse. What is altered, if the techniques are used correctly, is a visceral dislike of the beverage (i.e. its psychophysiological effect not merely its taste). Finally, and perhaps most important from the appropriate application of aversion therapies for excessive drinking can, at best, be but one part of an ensemble of therapies which will be needed to help a person with a serious alcohol problem back to a balanced life.

Acknowledgements
This work was supported, in part, by Grants NS 11618, AA03513-01A1, HD 05958, MCH 927, and DVS 49P-45192/9.

References

1. Harris MB. Self-directed program for control: a pilot study. J Abn Psychol 1969; 74: 263.
2. Edwards G, Orford J, Egert S et al. Alcoholism: a controlled trial of "treatment" and "advice". J Stud Alcohol 1977; 38: 1004–1031.
3. Kendell HE, Staton MC. The fate of untreated alcoholics. Q J Stud Alcohol 1965; 26: 685.
4. Elkins RL. Aversion therapy for alcoholism: chemical, electrical, or verbal. Int J Addict 1975; 10: 157.
5. Rachman SJ, Teasdale J. Aversion therapy and behaviour disorders: an analysis. Coral Gables: Univ of Miami Press, 1969.
6. Garcia J. Koelling RA. Relation of cue to consequence in avoidance learning. Psychon Sci 1966; 4: 123.
7. Garcia J, Hankins WG, Rusiniak K. Behavioural regulation of the milieu interne in man and rat. Science 1974; 185: 824.
8. Garcia J, Rusiniak KW, Brett LP. Conditioning food-illnesses aversions in wild animals: Caveant Canonici. In: Davis H, Hulvitz HMB, eds, Operant-Pavlovian interactions. New Jersey: Lawrence Erlbaum Association, 1977.
9. Garcia J, Hankins WG. The evolution of bitter and the acquisition of toxiphobia. In: Denton DA, Coughlan JP, eds. Olfaction and Taste, V. New York: Academic Press, 1975: 39–45.

10. Garcia J, Hankins WG. On the origin of food aversion paradigms. In: Hanker LM, Best MR, Domjan M. Learning mechanisms in food selection. Waco: Baylor Univ. Prss, 1977: 3–19.
11. Wilson GT, Davison GC. Aversion techniques in behaviour therapy: some theoretical and metatheoretical considerations. J Consult Clin Psychol 1969; 33: 327.
12. Lamon S, Wilson GT, Leaf RC. Human classical aversion conditioning: nausea versus electric shock in the reduction of large beverage consumption. Behav Res Ther. 1977; 15: 313.
13. Cannon DS, Baker TB and Wehl C. Emetic and electric shock alcohol aversion therapy. J Consult Clin Psychol 1981; 49: 360–368.
14. Bernstein IL. Learned taste aversions in children receiving chemotherapy. Science 1978; 200: 1302.
15. Rusiniak KG, Hankins WG, Garcia J, Brett LP. Flavour-illness aversions: potentiation of odor by taste in rats. Behav Biol 1978; in press.
16. Gustavson CR, Garcia J, Hankins WG, Rusiniak KW. Coyote predation control by aversive conditioning. Science 1974; 184: 581.
17. Gustavson CR, Kelly DJ, Sweeney M, Garcia J. Prey lithium aversions. I.: Coyotes and wolves. Behav Biol 1976; 17: 61.
18. Seligman MCP, Hager J, eds. Biological boundaries of learning. Englewood Cliffs, NJ: Prentice Hall, 1972.
19. Coil JD, Garcia J. Conditioned taste aversions: the illness US in biological approaches to learning. Papers presented at the Northeastern Regional Meeting of the Animal Behaviour Society, October 1977, St. Johns, Newfoundland. 1978.
20. Coil JD, Rodgers RC, Garcia J, Novin D. Conditioned taste aversions: vagal and circulating mediation of the toxic US. Behav Biol 1979; in press.
21. Borison HL, Wang SC. Physiology and pharmacology of vomiting. Pharmacol Rev 1953; 5: 193.
22. Garcia J, Ervin FR, Yorke CH, Koelling RA. Conditioning with delayed vitamin injection. Science 1967; 155: 716.
23. Maier SF, Zahorik DM, Albin RW. Relative novelty of solid and liquid diet during thiamine deficiency determines development of thiamine-specific hunger. J Comp Physiol Psychol 1971; 74: 254.

24. Green KH, Garcia J. Role of reinforcer in selecting and responding to cues. Proc. of the 78th Annual Convention of the American Psychological Association 1970; 1: 251.
25. Cabanac M. Physiological role of pleasure. Science 1971; 173: 1103.
26. Davis JD, Campbell CS. Peripheral control of meal size in the rat: effect of sham feeding on meal size and drinking rate. J Comp Physiol Psychol 1973; 83: 379.
27. Snowdon CT. Gastro-intestinal sensory and motor control of food intake. J Comp Physiol Psychol 1970; 71: 68.
28. Deutsch JA, Young WG, Kalogeris TJ. The stomach signals satiety. Science 1978; 201: 165.
29. Novin D, Gonzalez MF, Sanderson JD. Paradoxical increased feeding following glucose infusions in recovered lateral rats. Am J Physiol 1976; 230: 1084.
30. Rezek M, Novin D. Duodenal nutrient infusion: Effects on feeding in intact and vagotomized rabbits. J Nutr 1977; 106: 812.
31. Clarke JC, and Hayes K. Covert sensitization and the equipotentiality premise. Behav Res Ther 1984.
32. Mellor CS, White HP. Taste aversions to alcoholic beverages conditioned by motion sickness. Am J Psychiatry 1978; 135: 125.
33. Green L, Rachlin H. The effect of rotation on the learning of taste aversions. Bull Psychonomic Soc 1973; 1: 137.
34. Norgren R, Pfaffman C. The pontine taste area in the rat. Brain Res 1975; 91: 99.
35. Brett LP, Hankins WG, and Garcia J. Prey lithium aversions III. Buteo Hawks. Behav Biol 1976; 17: 87.
36. Clarke JC, Westbrook RF, Irwin J. Flavor-illness aversions: Potentiation of color by taste in pigeons. Behav Biol 1979; 25: 18–29.
37. Testa TJ, Ternes JW. Specificity of conditioning mechanisms in the modification of food preferences. In: Barker LM, Best MR, Domjan M, eds, Learning mechanisms in food selection. Waco: Baylor Univ. Press, 1977; 229–253.
38. Dietz MN, Carpetta PJ. Modification of sugar-saccharin preferences in rats as a function of electric shock to the mouth. Proceedings of the 74th Annual Convention of the American Psychological Association 1966; 1: 161.

39. Green L, Bouzas A, Rachlin H. Text of an electric shock analog to illness-induced aversion. Behav Biol 1972; 7:513.
40. Rusiniak KW, Garcia J, Hankins WG. Bait shyness: Avoidance of the taste without escape from the illness. J Comp Physiol Psychol 1976; 90: 460.
41. Kelly DJ. Facilitative effects of specific taste cues on odor aversion learning. Personal communication, Arizona State Univ. 1978.
42. Rusiniak KG. Bait shyness: Potentiation of weak odor by strong taste in adult and weaning rats. Paper presented at the Psychomic Society Meeting, San Antonio, Texas, 1978.
43. Lemere F, Voegtlin WL. An evaluation of the aversion treatment of alcoholism. Q J Stud Alcohol 1950; 11: 199.
44. Sanderson RE, Campbell D, Laverty SG. An investigation of a new aversive conditioning treatment for alcoholism. Q J Stud Alcohol 1963; 24: 261.
45. Revusky S, Gorry T. Flavor aversions produced by contingent injection: relative effectiveness of apomorphine, emetine, and lithium. Behav Res Ther 1973; 11: 403.
46. Revusky S. Some laboratory paradigms for chemical aversion treatment of alcoholism. J Behav Ther Exp Psychiatry 1973; 4: 15.

*Reprinted from *Australian Drug and Alcohol Review,* 1986, *5,* 21-27

APPENDIX C

Rationale-Emotive Therapy

Homework Sheets

As you fill in the details, recall that 'A' refers to the event (for example, finding you have a flat tyre, seeing friends going into a bottle shop), situation (for example, visiting relatives, meeting the person you work for, having an interview for a job) or outcome (for example, having an argument, doing badly in a job evaluation report) associated with a negative emotion 'C'. The letter 'B' refers to the beliefs, thoughts, mental images and self-talk in and after the occurrence of the 'A' condition. Your emotional reactions should be listed under 'C'. The letter 'D' refers to the use of 'reasonable' self-directions and self-evaluation with which to dispute or to challenge unreasonable interpretations and conclusions (the maladaptive 'B's). It is best to complete the A-B-C-D form as soon as possible after a distressing episode so that you will have the best chance of recalling problem-causing 'B' activities. If you cannot recall or detect any obvious ones put down your best guess as to what 'silent' or 'automatic' beliefs could have intervened between 'A' (the outside event, situation) and 'C' (your emotional reactions which occurred during 'A' or afterwards when you recalled what went on in the 'A' situation). Lastly, list what actions or thoughts you would attempt to use if another such 'A' occurs.

References

Chapter 1

1. P. Miller, *Behavioral treatment of alcoholism.* New York: Pergamon Press, 1976.
2. F. Baekeland, Evaluation of treatment methods in chronic alcoholism. In B. Kissin & H. Begleiter (Eds), *Treatment and rehabilitation of the chronic alcoholic.* New York: Plenum Press, 1977.
3. Ibid.
4. J. Kinney, & G. Leaton (Eds), *Understanding alcohol.* New York: New American Library, 1982.
5. Ibid.
6. Ibid.
7. Ibid.
8. Ibid.
9. J. Saunders, Changing perspectives on alcohol and drug problems. *Australian Drug and Alcohol Review,* 1986, *5,* 41–45.
10. A. Tyler, *Street drugs.* Kent: New English Library, 1986.
11. H. Blane, W. Overton & M. Chafetz, Social factors in the diagnosis of alcoholism. *Quarterly Journal of Studies in Alcoholism,* 1963, *26,* 640.
12. Ibid.
13. B. Hore, *Alcohol dependence.* London: Butterworths, 1976.
14. See 11.
15. M. Jacobs, *Problems presented by alcoholic clients.* Toronto: Addiction Research Foundation, 1981.
16. H. Trice, *Alcoholism in America.* New York: McGraw-Hill, 1966.
17. See 15.

Chapter 2

1. R. Strauss, Problem drinking in the perspective of social change. In W. Filstead (Ed.), *Alcohol and alcohol problems.* Cambridge, Mass: Ballinger, 1976.
2. Anonymous, *Alcoholics anonymous.* New York: Works Publishing, 1939.
3. Ibid.
4. W. Glaser, *Control therapy.* New York: Harper & Row, 1984.
5. L. Wolberg, *The technique of psychotherapy.* New York: Grune and Stratton, 1954.
6. J.G. Strachan. *Alcoholism: a treatable illness.* Vancouver: Mitchell

Press, 1982.
7. M.N. Weisman, letter in *News and Views*, newsletter published by the Alcoholism Council of Greater Los Angeles, January 1975.
8. E.M. Jellinek, *The disease concept of alcoholism*. New Brunswick, N.J.: Hillhouse Press, 1960.
9. Ibid.
10. M. Sanchez-Craig, personal communication.
11. A. Marlatt, B. Demming & J. Reid, Loss of control drinking in alcoholics: an experimental analogue. *Journal of Abnormal Psychology*, 1973, *81*, 233–241.
12. N. Heather & I. Robertson, *Controlled drinking*, London: Methuen, 1981.
13. J. Merry, The 'loss of control' myth. *Lancet*, 1966, 1, 1257–1258.
14. See 11.
15. P. Miller, *Behavioural treatment of alcoholism*. Oxford: Pergamon Press, 1976.

Chapter 3

1. P. Miller, *Behavioral treatment of alcoholism*. Oxford: Pergamon, 1976.
2. W. Miller, Controlled drinking: a history and a critical review. *Journal of Studies in Alcohol*, 1983, *44*, 68–82.
3. F. Baekeland, Evaluation of treatment methods in chronic alcoholism. In B. Kissin & H. Begleiter (Eds), *Treatment and rehabilitation of the chronic alcoholic*. New York: Plenum Press, 1977.
4. R. Costello, P. Biever & J. Baillargeon, Alcoholism treatment programmes. *Alcoholism Clinical and Experimental Research*, 1977, *1*, 311–318.
5. J. Helzer, L. Robins, J. Taylor, K. Carey, R. Miller, T. Combs-Orme & A. Farmer, The extent of long-term moderate drinking among alcoholics discharged from medical and psychiatric treatment facilities. *New England Journal of Medicine*, 1985, *126*, 1678–1682.
6. V. Fox, The controlled drinking controversy (editorial). *Journal of the American Medical Association*, 1976, 236, 863.
7. W. Miller, Controlled drinking: a history and a critical review. *Journal of Studies in Alcohol*, 1983, 44, 68–82.
8. Ibid.
9. D.L. Davies, Normal drinking in recovered alcohol addicts. *Quarterly Journal of Studies on Alcohol*, 1962, *23*, 94–104.
10. D. Armour, J. Polich & H.B. Stambul, *Alcoholism and treatment*. New

York: Wiley, 1978.
11. See 9.
12. R.E. Kendall & M.C. Stanton, The fate of untreated alcoholics. *Quarterly Journal of Studies on Alcohol*, 1966, *27*, 30–41.
13. S. Lovibond & G. Caddy, Discriminated aversive control in the moderation of alcoholics' drinking behaviour. *Behavior Therapy*, 1970, *1*, 437–444.
14. M. Sobell & L. Sobell, *Behavioral treatment of alcohol problems*. New York: Plenum Press, 1978.
15. M. Pendery, I. Maltzman & J. West, Controlled drinking by alcoholics? New findings and a reevaluation of a major affirmative study. *Science*, 1982, *217*, 169–175.
16. See 5.
17. E.M. Jellinek, *The disease concept of alcoholism*. New Brunswick, N.J.: Hillhouse Press, 1960.
18. Ibid.
19. G. Edwards, *The treatment of drinking problems*. New York: McGraw-Hill, 1982.
20. Ibid.
21. Ibid.
22. T.R. Stockwell, R. Hodgson, G. Edwards, C. Taylor & H. Rankin, The development of a questionnaire to measure severity of alcohol dependence. *British Journal of Addiction*, 1979, *74*, 79–87.
23. H. Skinner & B. Allen, Alcohol dependence syndrome. *Journal of Abnormal Psychology*, 1982, *91*, 199–208.
24. J. Orford, E. Oppenheimer & G. Edwards, Abstinence or control: the outcome for excessive drinkers two years after consultation. *Behaviour Research and Therapy*, 1976, *14*, 409–418.
25. J. Polich, D. Armour & Braiker H., Patterns of alcoholism over four years. *Journal of Studies on Alcohol*, 1980, *41*, 397–416.
26. A.D. Wodak, J.B. Saunders, I. Ewusi-Menash, M. Davies & R. Williams, Severity of alcohol dependence in patients with alcoholic liver disease. *British Medical Journal*, 1983, *287*, 1140–1143.
27. I. Robertson, Controlled drinking—an approach to management. *Australian Alcohol/Drug Review*, 1985, *4*, 257–266.
28. M. Sanchez-Craig, H. Annis, A. Bornet & K. MacDonald, Random assignment to abstinence and controlled drinking: evaluation of a cognitive-behavioural program for problem drinkers. *Journal of Consulting and Clinical Psychology*, 1984, *52* (*3*), 399–403.
29. D. Jolly, E. Fleece, A. Galanos, J. Milby and S. Ritter, DSM-III:

alcohol abuse and alcohol dependence: interrator diagnostic reliability. *Addictive Behaviors*, 1983, *8*, 201–204.

Chapter 4

1. M. Sobell & L. Sobell, *Behavioural treatment of alcohol problems*. New York: Plenum Press, 1978.
2. Ibid.
3. J.B. Saunders & R. Williams, The genetics of alcoholism: is there an inherited susceptibility to alcohol-related problems? *Alcohol and Alcoholism*, 1983, *18*, 189–217.
4. R.W. Hyde & L.V. Kingsley, Studies in medical sociology. *New England Journal of Medicine*, 1944, *231*, 543–548.
5. G.L. Muhlin, Ethnic differences in alcohol misuse: a striking reaffirmation. *Journal of Studies on Alcohol*, 1984, 172–173.
6. G. Crothers in V. Horsley (Ed.) *Alcohol and the human body*. New York: Macmillan, 1909.
7. See 3.
8. J. Neale & T. Oltmanns, *Schizophrenia*. New York: Wiley, 1980.
9. C.R. Snyder, Culture and Jewish sobriety—the in group-out group factor. In D.J. Pittman & C.R. Snyder (Eds), *Society, culture and drinking patterns*. New York: Wiley, 1962.
10. B. Caudill & G.A. Marlatt, Modeling influences in social drinking: an experimental analogue. *Journal of Consulting and Clinical Psychology*, 1975, *43*, 405–415.
11. R.L. Collins, G.A. Parks & G.A. Marlatt, Social determinants of alcohol consumption: the effects of social interaction and model status on the self-administration of alcohol. *Journal of Consulting and Clincial Psychology*. 1985, *53*, 189–200.
12. Ibid.
13. G.R. Jacobsen, An introduction to psychological factors in the etiology and treatment of alcoholism. In M. Galanter (Ed.), *Currents in alcoholism*. New York: Grune & Stratton, 1980.
14. H. Trice, *Alcoholism in America*. New York: McGraw-Hill, 1966.
15. A.R. Tarbox, Alcoholism, biofeedback and internal scanning. *Journal of Studies on Alcohol*, 1983, *44*, 246–261.
16. P. Nathan & J. O'Brien, An experimental analysis of the behavior of alcoholics and non alcoholics during prolonged experimental drinking. *Behavior Therapy*, 1971, *2*, 455–476.
17. N.K. Mello, Behavioural studies of alcoholism. In B. Kissin and H. Begleiter (Eds), *The biology of alcoholism*. New York: Plenum Press, 1972.

18. A. Paredes, Overview: psychological and treatment issues. In M. Galanter (Ed.), *Currents in alcoholism*. New York: Grune & Stratton, 1980.
19. J. Steffen, P. Nathan & H. Taylor, Tension-reducing effects of alcohol: further evidence and some methodological considerations. *Journal of Abnormal Psychology*, 1974, *5*, 547–547.
20. J.S. Tamerin, S. Weiner & J.H. Mendelson, Alcoholics' expectancies and recall of experiences during intoxication. *American Journal of Psychiatry*, 1970, *126*, 1697–1704.
21. J. Jaffe, Alcoholism and affective disturbance: current drugs and current shortcomings. In G. Edwards & J. Littleton (Eds), *Pharmacological treatments for alcoholism*. London: Croom-Helm, 1984.
22. B. Thyer, R. Parrish, J. Himle, O. Cameron, G. Curtis and R. Nesse, Alcohol abuse among clinically anxious patients. *Behaviour Research and Therapy*, 1986, *24*, 357–359.
23. P. Miller, M. Hersen, R. Eisler & G. Hilsman, Effects of social stress on operant drinking of alcoholics and social drinkers. *Behaviour Research and Therapy*, 1974, *12*, 67–72.
24. G.A. Marlatt & J.R. Gordon, *Relapse prevention*. New York: Guilford Press, 1985.

Chapter 5

1. D.J. Pittman & M.W. Sterne, A concept of motivation—a source of institutional blockage in the treatment of alcoholics. *Quarterly Journal of Studies on Alcohol*, 1965, *26*, 41–57.
2. Ibid.
3. R. Fox, Treatment of chronic alcoholism. *The Medical Clinics of North America*, 1958, *42*, 805–814.
4. R. Fox, A multidisciplinary approach to the treatment of alcoholism. *American Journal of Psychotherapy*, 1967, *123*, 769–778.
5. A. Moore, Alcholism treatment in private psychiatric hospitals: a national survey. *Quarterly Journal of Studies on Alcohol*, 1971, *32*, 1083–1085.
6. Alcoholics Anonymous, *Alcoholics Anonymous: the story of how many thousands of men and women have recovered from alcoholism*. New York: Alcoholics Anonymous, 1955.
7. R. Glasscote, T. Plaute, D.W. Hammersley, F.J. O'Neill, M. Chafetz & E. Cumming, *The treatment of alcoholism: a study of program and problems*. Washington: Joint Information Service, American Psychiatric Association and National Association for Mental Health, 1967.

8. A.A. Cavaiola, Resistance issues in the treatment of the DWI offender. *Alcoholism Treatment Quarterly*, 1984, *1*, 87–100.
9. W. Miller, Motivation for treatment: a review with special emphasis on alcoholism. *Psychological Bulletin*, 1985, *98*, 84–107.
10. R.S. Greenburger, Sobering method: firms are confronting alcoholic executives with threat of firing. *The Wall Street Journal*, 13 January 1983, pp.1, 26.
11. Ibid.
12. L. DiCicco, H. Unterberger & J. Mack, Confronting denial. *Psychiatric Annals*, 1978, *8*, 596–606.
13. M. Jacobs, *Problems presented by alcoholic clients*. Toronto: Addiction Research Foundation, 1981.
14. See 9.
15. W.C. Paneptino & M.J. Higgins, Keeping alcoholics in treatment: effective follow-through procedures. *Quarterly Journal of Studies on Alcohol*, 1969, *30*, 414–419.
16. See 13.
17. See 13.
18. A. Koumans, J. Muller and C. Miller, Use of telephone calls to increase motivation for treatment in alcoholics. *Psychological Reports*, 1967, *21*, 327–328.
19. G. Leake & A. King, Effect of counsellor expectations on alcoholic recovery. *Alcohol Health and Research World*, 1977, *11(3)*, 16–22.
20. See 9.
21. See 13.
22. G. Edwards, *The treatment of drinking problems*. New York: McGraw-Hill, 1982.

Chapter 6

1. A. Auerbach, Assessment of psychotherapy outcome from the viewpoint of the expert observer. In M. Lambert, E. Christensen & S. Dejulio (Eds) *The assessment of psychotherapy outcome*. New York: John Wiley, 1983.
2. P. Miller, *Behavioural treatment of alcoholism*. Oxford: Pergamon Press, 1976.
3. K.D. O'Leary, A. Curley, A. Rosenbaum & J.C. Clarke, Assertion training for wives: a potentially hazardous treatment? *Journal of Marital & Family Therapy*, 1985, Vol II No 3, 319–332.
4. G. Edwards, The treatment of drinking problems. New York: McGraw-Hill, 1982.

5. Ibid.
6. A. Beck, *Depression*. New York: Harper & Row, 1967.
7. A. Pokorny, B.A. Miller and H. Kaplan, The brief MAST: a shortened version of the Michigan Alcoholic Screening Test. *American Journal of Psychiatry*, 1972, *129*, 342–345.
8. D. Mayfield, G. McLeod & D. Hall, The CAGE questionnaire: validation of a new alcoholism screening instrument. *American Journal of Psychiatry*, 1974, *131*, 1121–1123.
9. M. McIntosh & M. Sanchez-Craig, Moderate drinking: a treatment goal for early stage problem drinking. *Canadian Medical Association Journal*, 1984, *131*, 873–876.
10. See 3.
11. M. Sanchez-Craig & Y. Israel, Pattern of alcohol consumption with self identified problem drinking. *American Journal of Public Health*, 1985, *75*, 175–180.
12. A. Lazarus, *Behaviour therapy and beyond*. New York: McGraw-Hill, 1971.
13. D. Cahalan, *Problem drinkers; a national survey*. San Francisco: Jossey-Bass, 1970.
14. M. Weissman, J. Myers & P. Harding, Prevalence and psychiatric heterogeneity of alcoholism in a U.S. urban community. *Journal of Studies in Alcohol*, 1980, *41*, 672–681.
15. D. Mayfield, Substance abuse in affective disorders. In A. Alterman (Ed.), *Substance abuse and psychopathology*. New York: Plenum Press, 1980.
16. A.D. Pokorny, The multiple readmission psychiatric patient. *Psychiatric Quarterly*, 1965, *39*, 70–78.
17. See 3.
18. See 3.
19. G.A. Marlatt & J.R. Gordon, *Relapse prevention*. New York: Guilford Press, 1985.
20. S. Shaw, The disease concept of dependence. In N. Heather, I. Robertson & D. Davies (Eds), *The misuse of alcohol*. New York: New York University Press, 1985.
21. H. Skinner & B. Allen, Alcohol dependence syndrome. *Journal of Abnormal Psychology*, 1982, *91*, 199–209.
22. Ibid.
23. T.R. Stockwell, R. Hodgson, G. Edwards, C. Taylor & H. Rankin, The development of a questionnaire to measure severity of alcohol dependence. *British Journal of Addiction*, 1979, *74*, 79–87.
24. R. Davidson & D. Raistrick, The validity of the short alcohol depen-

dence data (SADD). *British Journal of Addiction*, 1986, *81*, 217–222.
25. N. Heather, S. Rollnick and M. Winton, A comparison of objective and subjective measures of alcohol dependence as predictors of relapse following treatment. *British Journal of Clinical Psychology*, 1983, *22*, 11–17.
26. Ibid.
27. I. Grant & R. Reed, Neuropsychology of alcohol and drug abuse. In A. Alterman (Ed.), *Substance abuse and psychopathology*. New York: Plenum Press, 1980.
28. J. Polich, D. Armour & H. Braiker, Patterns of alcoholism over four years. *Journal of Studies on Alcohol*, 1980, *41*, 397–416.

Chapter 7

1. C.S. Lieber, *Medical complications of alcoholism*. Philadelphia, W.B. Saunders, 1981.
2. J.B. Saunders & O.G. Aasland. *WHO collaborative project on identification and treatment of persons with harmful alcohol consumption. Report on Phase I. Development of a screening instrument*. Geneva: World Health Organization, 1987.
3. H.A. Skinner, S. Holt, W.J. Sheu & Y. Israel, Clinical versus laboratory detection of alcohol abuse: the Alcohol Clinical Index. *British Medical Journal*, 1986, *292*, 1703–1708.
4. T. Stockwell, R. Hodgson, G. Edwards, C. Taylor & H. Rankin, The development of a questionnaire to measure severity of alcohol dependence. *British Journal of Addiction*, 1979, *74*, 79–87.

Chapter 8

1. J.B. Saunders, Drug treatment in alcoholism. In G.D. Burrows, T.R. Norman & B. Davies (Eds), *Antimanics, anticonvulsants and other drugs in psychiatry (Drugs in psychiatry, Volume 4)*. Amsterdam: Elsevier, 1987.
2. J.B. Saunders, Alcohol: an important cause of hypertension. *British Medical Journal*, 1987, *294*, 1045–1046.
3. G. Edwards & S. Guthrie. A controlled trial of inpatient and outpatient treatment of alcohol dependency. *Lancet*, 1967, *i*, 555–559.
4. G. Edwards, J. Orford, S. Guthrie, A. Hawker, C. Hensman, M. Mitchison, E. Oppenheimer & C. Taylor, Alcoholism: a controlled trial of 'treatment' and advice. *Journal of Studies on Alcohol*, 1977, *38*, 1004–1031.
5. H. Kristenson & B. Hood, The impact of alcohol on health in the general population: a review with particular reference to experience in

Malmo. *British Journal of Addiction*, 1984, *79*, 139–145.
6. J. Chick, G. Lloyd & E. Crombie, Counselling problem drinkers in medical wards: a controlled study. *British Medical Journal*, 1985, *290*, 965–967.
7. C.A. Naranjo, E.M. Sellers, J.T. Sullivan, D.V. Woodley, K. Kadlec & K. Sykora, The serotonin uptake inhibitor citalopram attenuates ethanol intake. *Clinical Pharmacology and Therapeutics*, 1987, *41*, 266–274.

Chapter 9

1. S. Rachman & J. Teasdale, *Aversion therapy: appraisal and status.* Coral Gables, Florida: University of Miami Press, 1969.
2. Ibid.
3. N. Hadley, *Foundations of aversion therapy.* New York: Spectrum, 1985.
4. Ibid.
5. See 1.
6. See 1.
7. J.C. Clarke & J. Garcia, Deranged ingestion: foundations of therapy for alcoholism. *Australian Drug and Alcohol Review*, 1986, *5*, 21–7.
8. J. Garcia, W.G. Hankins & J.D. Coil, Koalas, men and other conditioned gastronomes. In N. Milgram, L. Krames & T. Alloway (Eds), *Food aversion learning.* New York: Plenum Press, 1977.
9. Ibid.
10. J.C. Clarke, R.F. Westbrook & J. Irwin, Potentiation instead of overshadowing. *Behavioural and Neural Biology*, 1979, *25*, 18–29.
11. F. Le Mere & W. Voegtlin, An evaluation of the aversion treatment of alcoholism. *Quarterly Journal of Studies on Alcohol*, 1950, *17*, 199–204.
12. E.C. Miller, A. Dvorak & D.W. Turner, A method of creating aversion to alcohol by reflex conditioning in a group setting. *Quarterly Journal of Studies on Alcohol*, 1960, *21*, 424–431.
13. R. Elkins, Aversion therapy for alcoholism: chemical, electrical or verbal imaginary. *International Journal of Addictions*, 1975, *10*, 157–209.
14. A. Wiens & C. Menustik, Treatment outcome and patient characteristics in an aversion therapy program for alcoholism. *American Psychologist*, 1983, *38*, 1089–1096.
15. See 1.
16. See 7.

17. B. Blake, A follow-up of alcoholics treated by behavior therapy. *Behaviour Research and Therapy*, 1967, *5*, 89–94.
18. See 13.
19. R.E. Vogler, S.E. Lunde, G.R. Johnson & P.L. Martin, Electrical aversion conditioning with chronic alcoholics. *Journal of Consulting and Clinical Psychology*, 1970, *34*, 302–307.
20. A. Marlatt & J. Gordon, *Relapse prevention*. New York: Guilford Press, 1985.
21. See 7.
22. See 1.
23. R. Sanderson, D. Campbell & S. Laverty, An investigation of a new aversive conditioning technique for alcoholism. In C. Franks (Ed.), *Conditioning techniques in clinical practice and research*. New York: Springer, 1963.
24. See 7.
25. J.C. Clarke and W. Wardman, *Agoraphobia: a clinical and personal account*. Sydney: Pergamon, 1985.
26. See 7.
27. M. Seligman and J. Hager, *Biological boundaries and behavior*. New York: Appleton-Century-Crofts, 1972.
28. Ibid.
29. J. Cautela, Covert sensitization. *Psychological Reports*, 1967, *20*, 459–468.
30. J.C. Clarke and K. Hayes, Covert sensitization, stimulus relevance and the equipotentiality premise. *Behaviour Research and Therapy*, 1984, *22*, 451–454.

Chapter 10

1. D.O. Hebb, *The organization of behavior*. Philadelphia: Wiley, 1949.
2. O. Pomerlau, J. Fentig, L. Baker & N. Cooney, Reactivity to alcohol cues in alcoholics and nonalcoholics: Implications for a stimulus control analysis of drinking. *Addictive Behaviors*, 1983, *8*, 1–10.
3. A. Marlatt & J. Gordon, *Relapse prevention*. New York: Guilford Press, 1985.
4. Ibid.
5. M. Sanchez-Craig, D. Wilkinson & K. Walker, Theory and methods for secondary prevention of alcohol problems. In W. Cox (Ed.), *Treatment and prevention of alcohol problems*. New York: Academic Press, 1986.
6. G. Littman, Relapse in alcoholism. In. G. Edwards & M. Grant (Eds)

Alcoholism: treatment in transition. London: Croom Helm, 1980.
7. J.C. Clarke & J.A. Jackson, *Hypnosis and behavior therapy*. New York: Springer, 1983.
8. M. Goldfried & D. Sobocinski, The effect of irrational beliefs on emotional arousal. *Journal of Consulting and Clinical Psychology*, 1975, *43*, 504–510.
9. See 7.
10. A. Beck, A.J. Rush, B. Shaw & G. Emery, *Cognitive therapy of depression*. New York: Guilford Press, 1975.
11. P. Meehl, Schizotaxia, schizotypy, schizophrenia. *American Psychologist*, 1962, *17*, 827–838.
12. See 10.
13. T. Whalen, Wives of alcoholics. *Quarterly Journal of Studies on Alcohol*, 1953, *14*, 632–641.
14. G. Edwards, *The treatment of drinking problems*. New York: McGraw Hill, 1982.
15. J. Madden, *A guide to alcohol and drug dependence*. Bristol: Wright, 1984..i
16. S. Bok, *Lying*. New York: Anchor, 1984.
17. See 7.
18. J. Harwin, The excessive drinker and the family. In J. Orford & J. Harwin (Eds), *Alcohol and the family*. London: Croom Helm, 1982.
19. T. O'Farrell, H. Cutter & F. Floyd, Evaluating behavioral marital therapy for male alcoholics. *Behavior Therapy*, 1985, *16*, 147–167.
20. T. Gorski & M. Miller, *Counseling for relapse prevention*. Hazel Creste, Ill.: Alcoholism Systems Associates, 1979.

Chapter 11

1. A.R. Tarbox, Alcoholism, biofeedback and internal scanning. *Journal of Studies on Alcohol*, 1983, *44*, 246–261.
2. S. Brown, Expectancies versus background in the prediction of college drinking patterns. *Journal of Consulting and Clinical Psychology*, 1985, *53*, 123–130.
3. See 1.
4. See 1.
5. F. Klajner, L. Hartman and M. Sobell, Treatment of substance abuse by relaxation training. *Addictive Behaviors*, 1984, *9*, 41–55.
6. Ibid.
7. J.C. Clarke and J.A. Jackson, *Hypnosis and behavior therapy*. New York: Springer, 1983.
8. N. King, The therapeutic utility of abbreviated progressive relax-

ation: A critical review with implications for clinical practice. In M. Hersen, R.M. Eisler & P. Miller (Eds) *Progress in behavior modification*. New York: Academic Press, 1980.

9. T. Borkovec & J. Sides, Critical procedural variables related to the physiological effects of progressive relaxation: a review. *Behaviour Research and Therapy*, 1979, *17*, 119–125.
10. R. Lehrer & R.L. Woolfolk, Are stress-related techniques interchangeable or do they have special effects? in R.L. Woolfolk and R. Lehrer, *Handbook of relaxation and stress-reducing techniques*. New York: Guilford Press, 1983.
11. D.C. Rimm & J.C. Masters, *Behavior therapy*. New York: Academic Press, 1979.
12. H.S. Terrace, Stimulus control. In W. Honig (Ed.), *Operant behavior: areas of research and application*. New York: Appleton-Century-Crofts, 1966.
13. R.B. Malmo, *On emotions, needs, and our archaic brain*. New York: Holt, Rinehart & Winston, 1975.
14. Ibid.
15. See 10.
16. R.K. Russell & J.F. Sipich, Cue-controlled relaxation. *Journal of Behavior Therapy and Experimental Psychiatry*, 1973, *4*, 47–49.
17. D. Meichenbaum & D. Tuck, The cognitive-behavioral management of anxiety, anger and pain. In P. Davidson (Ed.), *The behavioral management of anxiety, depression and pain*. New York: Bruner/Mazel, 1976.
18. P. Lehrer, R.L. Woolfolk, A.J. Rooney, B. McGann & P. Carrington, Progressive relaxation and meditation. *Behaviour Research and Therapy*. 1983, *21*, 651–662.
19. H. Benson, *The relaxation response*. New York: William Morrow, 1975.
20. See 19.
21. B.C. Glueck & C. Stroebel, Biofeedback and meditation in the treatment of psychiatric illness. *Comprehensive Psychiatry*, 1975, *16*, 303–321.
22. D.S. Holmes, Medication and reduction in somatic arousal: a review of the experimental evidence. *American Psychologist*, 1984, *39*, 1–10.
23. E. Herrigel, *Zen in the art of archery*. New York: Pantheon Books, 1953.
24. See 12.
25. W. James, *The principles of psychology*, (Vol. 1), 1890.
26. See 20.

27. See 8.

Chapter 12.

1. W.A. Hunt, L.W. Barnett & L.G. Branch, Relapse rates in addiction programs. *Journal of Clinical Psychology*, 1971, *27*, 455–466.
2. I. Faloon, J. Boyd, C. McGill, J. Razani, H. Moss & A. Gilderman, Family management in the prevention of exacerbation of schizophrenia: a controlled study. *New England Journal of Medicine*, 1982, *306*, 1437–1440.
3. C. Cummings, J. Gordon & G. Marlatt, Relapse: strategies of prevention and prediction. In W. Miller (Ed.), *The addictive behaviors*. Oxford: Pergamon Press, 1980.
4. G. Littman, Relapse in alcoholism. In G. Edwards & M. Grant (Eds) *Alcoholism: treatment in transition*. London: Croom Helm, 1980.
5. P. Meehl, Schizotaxia, schizotypy, schizophrenia. *American Psychologist*, 1962, *17*, 827–838.
6. E. Chaney, M. O'Leary & G. Marlatt, Skill training with alcoholics. *Journal of Consulting and Clinical Psychology*, 1978, *46*, 1092–1104.
7. H. Rankin, R. Hodgson & T. Stockwell, Cue exposure and response prevention with alcoholics. *Behaviour Research and Therapy*, 1983, *21*, 435–446.
8. R. Hodgson & H. Rankin, Cue exposure and relapse prevention. In W. Hay and P. Nathan (Eds), *Clinical case studies in the behavioral treatment of alcoholism*. New York: Plenum Press, 1982.
9. O. Pomerleau, J. Fertig, L. Baker & N. Cooney, Reactivity to alcohol cues in alcoholics and non-alcoholics. *Addictive Behaviors*, 1983, *8*, 1–10.
10. B. Leach & J. Norris, Factors in the development of Alcoholics Anonymous. In B. Kissin & H. Begleiter (Eds), *Treatment and rehabilitation of the chronic alcoholic*. New York: Plenum Press, 1977.
11. G. Edwards, *The treatment of drinking problems*. New York: McGraw-Hill, 1982.
12. E.F. Torrey, *Witchdoctors and psychiatrists: the common roots of psychotherapy and its future*. New York: Harper & Row, 1986.

Index